The **Trustee** Handbook for Health Care Governance

The **Trustee** Handbook

for

HEALTH CARE

GOVERNANCE

JAMES E. ORLIKOFF
AND MARY K. TOTTEN

American Hospital Publishing, Inc.
An American Hospital Association Company
Chicago

American Hospital Publishing, Inc., gratefully acknowledges the financial support of Witt/Kieffer · Ford · Hadelman · Lloyd for the initial development of these materials.

Library of Congress Cataloging-in-Publication Data

Orlikoff, James E.
    The trustee handbook for health care governance / James E. Orlikoff and Mary K. Totten.
    p.   cm.
    A collection of articles that appeared in the magazine Trustee.
    1. Hospitals—Administration. 2. Hospital trustees. I. Totten, Mary K. II. American Hospital Association. III. Trustee. IV. Title.
RA971.072 1998   97-31677
362.1'1'068—dc21   CIP

ISBN: 1-55648-220-5   Item Number: 196140

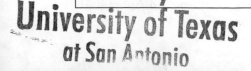

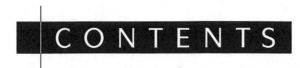
CONTENTS

ABOUT THE AUTHORS

James E. Orlikoff is president of Orlikoff & Associates, a Chicago-based consulting firm specializing in health care leadership, quality, and risk management. He was formerly the director of the American Hospital Association's Division of Hospital Governance and director of the Institute on Quality of Care and Patterns of Practice of the AHA's Hospital Research and Education Trust.

Mr. Orlikoff has been involved in quality, leadership, and risk management issues for over 10 years. He has designed and implemented hospital quality assurance and risk management programs in four countries and, since 1985, has worked with hospital governing boards to strengthen their overall effectiveness and their oversight of quality assurance and medical staff credentialing. He has written 6 books and over 40 articles and currently serves on hospital and civic boards.

Mary K. Totten is president of Totten & Associates, an Oak Park, Illinois–based consulting firm specializing in health care leadership. She was formerly program director for the Division of Hospital Governance of the American Hospital Association.

Ms. Totten has been a speaker and consultant to hospital and system boards, hospital associations, and managed care organizations on strategic planning and mission development, quality of care, medical staff credentialing, governance restructuring, and other governance issues. She has managed grant projects; published monographs, briefing papers, and articles for hospital trustees; and has worked with national trustee leaders to assess the governing board's responsibility for quality care. She has also developed discussion forums and publications on defining and measuring quality for health care purchasers and providers.

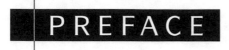

PREFACE

Revolutionary forces are buffeting the American health care system. These forces are challenging and profoundly changing American health care organizations. Yet, in the midst of all this revolutionary change, an important factor remains: effective health care organizations require effective governance. In fact, the more challenging the environment, the greater the pressures on a health care organization and the more effective a board must be.

Governance must rise to the occasion to be at peak effectiveness in order to lead an organization through this revolution. Unfortunately, just at a time when effective governance is more important than ever before, there is trouble in many boardrooms. Some boards intuitively realize that they are not up to the task before them and shy away from it. Others courageously attempt to confront the issues and find they are unable to do so because of weakness in the foundations of governance, lack of proper focus, lack of proper information and tools, or ineffective relationships with other leadership groups.

Not only must an effective board lead an organization through revolutionary change, it must also have the skills, tools, and determination to change itself. The emerging forms of health care organization require new forms of more focused governance to lead them.

Twelve "Trustee Workbooks," originally published in *Trustee* magazine, were designed to address the complex constellation of effective governance one issue at a time. They are reprinted as chapters of this book to provide a comprehensive and practical reference for and road map to effective governance. These chapters are organized in four sections, with each section of the book consisting of three chapters that relate to a common theme of effective governance.

The first section provides a primer on the foundations of effective governance. The basics of good governance are often predicated upon a board asking itself a series of structured questions. Such questions include the following:

- What talents, skills, experiences, and other attributes ought we to look for in the trustees we ask to serve on our governing boards?
- What are the basic roles and responsibilities of the board and of its individual members?
- Do we have a process in place to ensure that new board members, and from time-to-time our seasoned trustees, truly understand their governance responsibilities and the industry and organization in which they govern?

The first section, "Boardroom Basics," presents three interactive chapters designed to help boards answer these questions in ways that are meaningful to their process of governance and to the organizations they simultaneously lead and serve. Together, "Board Composition and Trustee Selection," "Board Job Descriptions," and "Orientation: Basic Building Blocks of Effective Boards" begin at the beginning to help boards build a solid foundation for effective governance.

The second section of this book, "Board Accountability," presents three interactive chapters that are designed to examine the most important aspects of board accountability. This section provides a framework to ensure continuously improved performance in serving both the organization and the community. "Board Accountability" enables boards to help steer their organizations to success by helping them

- to assess the health status of their community, commit to its improvement, and form alliances with other community leaders to develop a systems approach to a more accessible form of health care
- to create an organization-specific definition of quality that is measurable and drives development of meaningful strategies for quality improvement

- to use the board self-evaluation process to develop a team approach that improves the board's ability to govern and provides a model for the pursuit of excellence for the entire organization

Together, "Assessing and Improving Your Community's Health," "Board Oversight of Quality," and "Self-Evaluation: Mark of Good Governance" can help boards to guide themselves and their organizations toward excellence.

The third section introduces chapters that are intended to help focus a board on the organization's purpose, its strategy, and the information that the board needs to lead the organization through the process of change into the future. These chapters push a board to ask itself these critical questions:

- Is our mission statement clear, current, and applicable to our organization's capabilities?
- Do our strategic plan and the tactics that express it flow directly from our mission?
- How can we ensure that the information we receive supports our efforts to operate most effectively as the stewards of our health care organization's mission and strategic plan?

These three chapters focus boards on the critical areas of strategic planning and information. Together, "Developing a Community-Focused Mission," "Strategic Planning by the Board," and "Information and the Effective Board" can help boards clarify their fiduciary and social roles and guide the actualization of the organization's overall mission.

The final section of *The* Trustee *Handbook for Health Care Governance* examines the complex relationships that form the essence of an American health care organization. "Board Relations," reviews how a board must conceptualize and govern the critical relationships with the organization's CEO, physicians, and physician leaders.

The three chapters in this section, "CEO Evaluation and Compensation," "New Relationships with Physicians: An Overview for Trustees," and "The Board-Physician Partnership: Enhancing Leadership Potential," look at critical board relationships and discuss how to cultivate connections that are constructive and prosperous. These chapters will help trustees to consider

- how the board can help strengthen its relationship with the CEO and create a system of development, evaluation, and feedback that is clear, timely, and emphasizes consistency with the organization's mission
- what the variety of relationships are that organizations have with physicians and physician groups and how the board can oversee these relationships to ensure that they appropriately distribute risk, control costs, and still deliver quality care
- how the board can build a strong leadership partnership with the physicians associated with the organization

Each of the chapters in all four sections explores its topic in a format designed to engage board members in applying the issues and concepts to their own governance process. Every chapter begins with an overview of the topic, followed by discussion questions, exercises that help boards apply the material to their own situation, tips for improving governance effectiveness, and finally a topic-specific self-assessment questionnaire to help boards determine their own strengths and weaknesses and identify areas for improvement.

The Trustee *Handbook for Health Care Governance* can be used in a variety of ways and settings by the full board, board committees, or multidisciplinary leadership groups. For example, specific chapters could be used to explore a topic during time set aside for board education in conjunction with a regular board meeting or at a board retreat. The governance or board development committee of a board could use the entire book to help it plan and discharge its responsibilities for board member recruitment, orientation, and board development. Various other board committees, such as the board quality committee, the board executive committee, or the board strategic planning committee, could use the specific chapters relating to the topics of quality, CEO evaluation, and strategic planning to help perform their roles. Finally, this book can be used as part of a board self-evaluation to help assess and improve overall board performance.

This book will also be useful to individual board members who wish to examine a particular topic, to assess the function of the board, or to develop suggestions to improve certain aspects of governance. Thus, some exercises in each chapter can be completed by individual board members and the results shared with the full group as part of a planning or education session, to maximize the time available for thoughtful interaction among board members, or to develop board members individually.

We sincerely hope that *The* Trustee *Handbook for Health Care Governance* proves to be a key source of useful information for you and provides a key to opening the door to truly effective governance.

James E. Orlikoff and Mary K. Totten

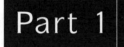

Part 1

Boardroom Basics

Board Composition and Trustee Selection

Immediately after making a speech to a group of film students about his work, director John Huston was cornered by a critical student. "Mr. Huston, do you realize that at least 50 percent of the success of your films is simply due to good casting?" the student rudely asserted. Unflappable, Huston replied, "My boy, my films are *100 percent* good casting."

The moral of the story? John Huston was a great director partially because he realized that the cast he chose could make or break a film. The same can be said for a governing board: The members of the board, why and how they are chosen, and how their skills and backgrounds are balanced to complement one another will have a huge impact on the effectiveness of that board and the success of the organization it governs.

When hospitals were in a relatively stable environment, the demands upon and contributions required of a board were predictable. Boards were homogeneous and stable and rarely had limits on terms of office, so trustee selection was an infrequent activity.

But in today's environment, boards need to start considering many other factors, including

- size
- criteria for selecting and recruiting new members
- criteria for reappointing trustees to additional terms
- establishing terms and term limits
- establishing policies and procedures to address ongoing trustee recruitment and other board functions

- establishing a board committee structure to perform these functions

Board Size

The proper size of a board depends on its roles and responsibilities. Nevertheless, the trend toward streamlining illustrates the emerging view that boards of fewer than 20 members tend to be more efficient.

Research suggests that the upper limit for effective and efficient group decision making is around 20 people. Anything larger can cause problems with communication and coordination, as well as the formation of factions and the diffusion of individual responsibility. The minimum size of a board depends on the number of members needed to provide a range of knowledge, skills, and experience.

Exercise: Board Size

Please read the following statements and answer the questions that follow. This exercise may be completed by individual trustees, then discussed with the entire board.

Following are arguments in favor of larger boards—those with more than 20 members:

- increased ability to represent all segments of the community and the organization's constituencies
- ability to spread the work among more members
- ability to recruit affluent and politically connected people who will not participate in board functions other than raising funds and conducting political advocacy activities

Following are some arguments against larger boards:

- more cumbersome decision making
- less commitment and involvement on the part of board members
- increased chance of "cliques" forming or power becoming vested in a subgroup of the board

Following are some arguments in favor of smaller boards—ones of 10 members or fewer:

- faster decision making
- more focus
- more flexibility
- fewer problems with communication and coordination

Following are some arguments against small boards:

- burnout as a result of trustees being spread too thin on board and committee work
- difficulty of achieving a good mix of skills, knowledge, and experience
- potential lack of depth if there is unexpected trustee turnover
- potential ability of one or two individuals to exert a disproportionate influence on the board's decisions

1. Which of the preceding arguments do and your board find more persuasive?
2. How large is your board? Is this size appropriate?
3. Why is your board this size?
4. Should the size of your board be modified? If so, how?

Who Should Be on the Board?

Obviously, the makeup of the board affects its function, so trustees should be chosen carefully. Further, the choice of members should be based on some type of criteria that takes into account the board's needs as well as the likely contributions of potential members.

But many boards do not have clearly articulated functions, so asking who should serve is putting the cart before the horse. Before trustees can be selected, the board as a whole needs to decide: What are we supposed to do? What individual skills, characteristics, and backgrounds of people will most effectively allow the board to do its job?

This progression is logical, but it's seldom simple. That's because most boards have many functions, some explicit, some implicit. Each function places different, and frequently contradictory, demands on board composition.

If a board is supposed to represent the community, for example, some would say that its membership should be a cross section of the community. If the board is supposed to exercise business acumen, that argues for trustees with business expertise. Trustees with backgrounds in health care may contribute to the board's function, but so might trustees with legal, accounting, or social service backgrounds, and so on.

Questions for Discussion

1. Why is your board composed as it currently is?
2. Why were you chosen to be a member?
3. Is the current makeup of the board ideal for addressing the changing issues, trends, and threats in health care?
4. As you survey the board, what skills are missing that will be needed to address the changing health care environment?
5. How many of your trustees are members of your organization's defined community? Is that number appropriate?
6. How is your governing board's composition different today than it was five years ago?
7. How will your board's composition likely be different five years from now?

Tips for Effective Governance Composition and Trustee Selection

- Clarify and articulate the board's functions and make them the foundation for the development of criteria for new trustee selection.
- Translate the functions of the board into a written job description that states roles and responsibilities.
- Develop a written trustee job description and use it as the basis for developing performance criteria to determine trustee reappointment.
- Establish a structured, integrated, and specific system of trustee selection, reappointment, and board composition.

- Develop a profile containing each board member's key characteristics, such as skills, experience, and background, in order to help identify gaps or areas of need on the board.
- Institute term limits for members of the board (for example, a three-year term with a maximum of three consecutive terms for a total of nine years of possible consecutive board membership).
- Systematically employ criteria for reappointment that assess all board members. Trustee terms should not be renewed automatically.
- Make the board a workable size—between 10 and 20 members.
- Assign responsibility to a board development or nominating committee to develop an integrated approach to trustee selection, reappointment, and board composition.
- Link the development of criteria for selecting new trustees to the annual board objectives, the work plan, and the organization's strategic plan.
- Annually evaluate the process, criteria, and priorities used to select and reappoint trustees and balance board composition.

Credentialing Trustees: A Future Trend?

As integrated delivery systems (IDSs) emerge, questions arise about the leadership skills, big-picture thinking, and political savvy necessary to effectively govern them. Some wonder if billion-dollar health systems should be governed by "amateur" trustees.

Doctors need credentialing before they can be appointed and reappointed to a medical staff, managed care panel, or physician-hospital organization (PHO). Will the trustees of tomorrow's IDSs and health care organizations need to be credentialed as well? Futurists like Russell C. Coile Jr. think so.

In the future, health systems may set very explicit criteria for system board membership. One such criterion could be past governance experience, according to evidence from a long-range study of nine IDSs.

This research study, conducted by Stephen Shortell, Ph.D., of Northwestern University, suggests that successful systems are governed by trustees who have already had experience at the hospital or other institutional board level.

Credentialing Criteria for Board Membership

Possible categories of criteria for member selection and reappointment include general qualifications criteria, demographic criteria, specific qualifications criteria, and position criteria.

Because all trustees must meet the general qualifications criteria, these should be applied fairly rigidly. For example, there is no point in selecting an otherwise wonderful trustee who cannot attend a majority of meetings, participate in group decision making, or keep confidential matters confidential.

Demographic criteria relate to such issues as the geographic location of board members, as well as the age, gender, and racial mix of the board. Typically, demographic criteria are used as flexible guidelines rather than rigid rules.

Specific qualifications criteria should reflect both the continuing and specific needs of a well-rounded board. It is in this category that knowledge, skills, experience, occupation, contacts, politics, affluence, and other characteristics are employed. Specific qualifications criteria are typically used to create a balance of skills, experience, and knowledge.

Finally, position criteria establish membership positions for individuals who hold specific jobs, usually within the organization. A typical example is a bylaws requirement that grants ex-officio membership (with voting power) to the hospital CEO and the chief of the medical staff.

Exercise: Trustee Selection Criteria

---

1. Please review the following sets of criteria, then rank those that would be most important when establishing an effective board for a health care organization of tomorrow. This may be done individually, then discussed with the entire board.
   - general qualifications criteria
     —willingness to serve on the hospital board
     —ability to meet the projected time commitment
     —ability to function as a member of a deliberative body

—willingness to undergo board orientation and continuing education
—objectivity
—intelligence
—communication skills
—integrity and the absence of conflict of interest
—values

- demographic criteria
  —Should all trustees be required to live within certain geographical boundaries?
  —Should at least one trustee serve on the board who does not live in the organization's service area?
  —Should there be age parameters for membership (for example, a minimum age of 21 and a maximum of 75)?
  —Should an attempt be made to balance board membership on the basis of gender?
  —Should an attempt be made to balance board membership on the basis of race?

- specific qualifications criteria
  —prior experience on other boards (such as membership on the board of a hospital with at least 300 beds, a system with $50 million to $100 million in combined revenues, or a 50-plus physician medical group practice; or at least three years on the board of a large private-sector corporation or not-for-profit organization)
  —professional and business achievements
  —specific occupation and skills, such as business, medicine, law, or nursing
  —leadership skills
  —big-picture skills
  —systems thinking skills
  —a record of community involvement and commitment
  —political connections
  —experience in mergers in other organizations
  —experience in downsizing in other organizations
  —experience in reengineering in other organizations
  —experience as an executive or board member of a major health care purchaser (such as a large employer or local or county government)

- position criteria
  —health care organization CEO
  —other health care organization senior executives
  —president of the PHO
  —chair of the PHO board
  —chair of the foundation
  —chair of the auxiliary
2. Should criteria for reappointment to the board for additional terms be developed and used by the nominating or board development committee? Such criteria could include
   - minimum attendance requirements for board meetings
   - regular attendance at board committee meetings
   - meaningful participation at board and committee meetings
   - preparation in advance for meetings
   - attendance at a set minimum of board continuing education sessions
3. What other criteria or categories of criteria for board membership should be considered?

Board Profiling for Effective Composition and Trustee Selection

To get a picture of your board's profile, develop a chart that outlines the skills, qualifications, demographic characteristics, and tenure of each trustee. Use the chart or profile to identify gaps in the board—such as missing or redundant expertise or demographic characteristics.

You can then develop a profile of the characteristics and composition of an ideal board. Obviously, no one ideal board for all health care organizations exists. But the ideal can be compared with the profile of your current board, and differences between the two can form the basis for developing criteria for selecting and reappointing trustees.

Exercise: Board Profiling

1. Develop a profile of your board. For each member, list expertise, areas of interest, professional background, type and length of community involvement, age, residency, gender,

race, ethnicity, board tenure, and years remaining until the maximum term limit is reached. Now consider the following:

- What are the areas of duplication or member clustering on the board? (For example, it may be composed of a majority of white, 60-year-old bankers, with two years left until they reach the maximum term limit.)
- What are the demographic characteristics that are underrepresented on the board?
- Based on the board profile, what characteristics should be sought in the next three trustees you recruit?

2. Develop a profile of the "ideal" board for helping your organization achieve its strategic plan.

3. Compare your current board profile with your ideal. What differences exist between the two? Based upon these differences, what criteria for new trustee selection should your board develop and employ? What criteria for trustee reappointment should you develop or discard?

Board Composition and Trustee Selection: A Self-Assessment Questionnaire

The following survey addresses the board's responsibilities in selecting its own members and maintaining a proper trustee composition. It can be used as a stand-alone survey or as part of an overall board self-evaluation. Have each trustee independently and anonymously rate performance on the following questions. Compile and analyze all the responses and discuss them with the entire board. The discussion should result in an action plan to improve performance.

1. The current size of our board is appropriate and contributes to efficient and effective board performance.

   ❑ Strongly Agree   ❑ Agree
   ❑ Somewhat Disagree   ❑ Disagree

2. Bylaws determine our board's size.

   ❑ Strongly Agree   ❑ Agree
   ❑ Somewhat Disagree   ❑ Disagree

3. Board members are selected based on preestablished criteria.

   ❑ Strongly Agree   ❑ Agree
   ❑ Somewhat Disagree ❑ Disagree

4. The board effectively identifies community leaders as potential new board members.

   ❑ Strongly Agree   ❑ Agree
   ❑ Somewhat Disagree ❑ Disagree

5. We limit the tenure of our board members to focus commitment and gain new expertise.

   ❑ Strongly Agree   ❑ Agree
   ❑ Somewhat Disagree ❑ Disagree

6. Reappointment depends on a review of the trustee's performance and is based on preestablished criteria.

   ❑ Strongly Agree   ❑ Agree
   ❑ Somewhat Disagree ❑ Disagree

7. A particular committee oversees the process for selecting and reappointing trustees.

   ❑ Strongly Agree   ❑ Agree
   ❑ Somewhat Disagree ❑ Disagree

8. When considering composition, we compare a profile of an ideal board with a profile of current members to identify needs, gaps, and redundancy.

   ❑ Strongly Agree   ❑ Agree
   ❑ Somewhat Disagree ❑ Disagree

9. Our board is properly composed to lead us into the 21st century and to achieve our strategic plan.

   ❑ Strongly Agree   ❑ Agree
   ❑ Somewhat Disagree ❑ Disagree

Conclusion

The members of the board, who they are, why they are chosen, whether they are reappointed to successive terms of office, all affect the function and effectiveness of the board and, ultimately, the organization.

As the health care environment changes, so does the character and function of governance. So, too, should the process of and criteria for selecting new board members.

Board Job Descriptions

There is one thing all boards have in common . . . they do not function.

—*Peter F. Drucker*

Tasks, Responsibilities, Practices

If we are unable to adequately describe what boards do, then how can we possibly hope to assess how well they do it?

—*Jeffrey A. Alexander, Ph.D., University of Michigan*

A health care governance consultant was asked recently, "If you could recommend only one thing to improve the performance of boards, what would it be?" Without hesitation he replied: "Job descriptions for boards, board members, and board leaders."

Why job descriptions? Because an extremely common cause of governance ineffectiveness is confusion among board members about what their roles and responsibilities are. Further, there is often confusion about the board's roles and responsibilities in relation to those of management, the medical staff, and other physician organizations; other boards; and committees of the board. Moreover, it is frequently unclear what the jobs of the board chair, committee chair, and board member are.

The most fundamental characteristic of excellent governance is that all board members have a shared understanding of their job. Every board has a somewhat different definition and allocation of its roles and responsibilities. Every board has a different mix of skills, personalities, and challenges. Every board must answer for itself the basic question: What is the job of the board of this health care organization?

The Purpose of Board Job Descriptions

Board job descriptions serve several important purposes, including

- *New board member recruitment:* Written board job descriptions help to focus the search for new trustees on individuals with the skills and talents that are most appropriate to the functions and needs of a board. More important, a well-written and up-to-date job description will let candidates know precisely what will be expected of them should they choose to join the board. Further, the job description tells potential candidates who have served on other boards the ways in which this one is unique.
- *New board member orientation:* A good position description details the role and work of the board and its members. This helps new members to become oriented more quickly and completely, to ask more informed questions, and to become more effective trustees.
- *Board self-evaluation:* Meaningful board self-evaluations are based upon a review of the effective discharge of the duties and responsibilities of the board. Thus, a board job description, along with annual board goals and objectives, provides a foundation for evaluating board performance.
- *Keeping governance on track:* A board job description allows board members to point out when a board is drifting away from performing some of its key roles and responsibilities. Further, it enables the board members to fine-tune the group's performance on an ongoing basis by comparing what the job description says the board should be doing with what it actually is doing.
- *Preventing conflict among multiple boards:* More than half of all U.S. health care organizations are part of

corporate structures that have more than one board. Job descriptions help prevent conflict among multiple boards (for example, disputes about which board has the authority to do what) as well as decision-making gridlock (where decisions cannot be made without the approval of each board, creating inappropriately long decision-cycle times).

- *Clarifying the practical distinction between governance and management:* An effective board-CEO relationship, one that is framed by a mutual understanding of relative roles and responsibilities, is vital to the success of the health care organization. Unfortunately, this key relationship is often framed by implicit assumptions about relative roles, expectations, and job functions. A board job description (along with a CEO job description) helps both sides to understand and respect the limits of each other's responsibilities, as well as to identify areas of joint responsibility.

Questions for Discussion

1. If your board has a job description, which of the above purposes are achieved by it? Which are not? Why?
2. If your board doesn't have a job description, why not? What other mechanisms are used to clarify the board's roles and responsibilities? Are these mechanisms effective?

Governance Roles and Responsibilities

The terms *roles* and *responsibilities* are often used interchangeably when describing the job of a board; there is, however, a difference. *Responsibilities* refers to what a board does or should do; *roles* refers to how the board does it. A meaningful job description should first outline the primary responsibilities of the board and then review the roles of the board in discharging those responsibilities. While roles, or how a board accomplishes its duties, will vary, the first step in creating a meaningful job description is to achieve agreement on the board's most important responsibilities.

Exercise: Potential Board Responsibilities

Consider the following potential board responsibilities, then answer the questions that follow. The board

- defines and pursues the mission and safeguard the values of the organization
- selects, monitors, supports, evaluates, and compensates the CEO
- establishes long-term direction through oversight of and participation in strategic planning
- promotes financial viability via budget and financial oversight, fund development, and investment management
- maintains and continuously improves the quality of care and services of the organization
- monitors the effectiveness of significant organizational programs and takes action where appropriate to improve, modify, or eliminate such programs as necessary to maintain organizational excellence
- oversees and promotes positive relationships with the medical staff and physician organizations
- promotes and maintains positive external relationships with the community, local business, government, funding sources, and other health-related organizations
- assures that the health care organization meets regulatory, accreditation, and legal requirements
- oversees effective governance, including trustee recruitment, selection, and orientation; board education and self-evaluation; and effective function and structure
- acts with the highest integrity to advance the best interests of the organization and achieve its mission
- represents the community
- oversees philanthropic fund-raising and participates in fund development through contributions
- sets policies for the organization
- serves as adviser to the CEO
- is an advocate for and provides links to specific constituent groups
- appoints and reappoints physicians to the medical staff and delineates their privileges
- represents the interests of the sponsoring religious order or owner

Questions for Discussion

1. Of these governance responsibilities, which are most important? Why?
2. Are there any governance responsibilities that are not mentioned above that you believe are important? Identify them and add them to the list.
3. If you were to choose only five of the above responsibilities to form the basis of a job description for your board, which would you pick? Why?
4. Make sure that all the members of your board, or the members of the committee charged with drafting a job description for your board, answer question 3. Did they all choose the same responsibilities? If yes, you have the basis of the job description for your board. If not, which were chosen most often? This should form the basis of a board discussion as you develop a board job description.
5. What role should the board play in discharging each of its responsibilities? For example, should the board initiate, lead, or respond to a given situation? Will the board discharge its quality oversight responsibility as a committee of the whole or use a committee to review such issues as physician credentialing or the use of quality indicators and make recommendations to the full governing board?

Exercise: Board Job Description

Below are three summaries of actual board job descriptions. Review them and then answer the questions that follow.

Memorial Hospital Board Job Description

Primary objective: The board is responsible for the success of the organization—both the quality of care and financial viability.
   Governance responsibilities:

- adopt the mission and determine the scope of services to be offered
- approve long-range plans
- select, support, and advise the CEO

- establish and maintain procedures for effective governance, including board member selection, orientation, education, and self-evaluation
- assure that quality care is provided and oversee the medical staff credentialing process
- serve as an advocate for the hospital in the community

General Hospital Board Job Description

The board's primary responsibility is to develop and follow the mission. This involves development and oversight of policy in four vital areas:

1. quality and performance improvement
2. financial performance
3. effective planning
4. effective management performance

To accomplish these responsibilities, the board

- establishes policy guidelines for mission implementation and achievement, as well as mission evaluation
- evaluates proposals to ensure that they are consistent with the mission
- monitors existing programs and activities of the hospital to ensure that they are consistent with the mission
- periodically reviews and, if necessary, revises the mission to ensure that it is relevant to the changing environment

Community Hospital Board Job Description

The board provides governance oversight for programmatic and policy-related aspects of all hospital services and corporate activities consistent with the Articles of Incorporation. The board also appoints the CEO and approves all actions that the executive committee takes in the name of the board between meetings.

Further, the board adopts and adheres to statements of mission, vision, strategy, and values that are reviewed on a regular basis. It considers the health requirements of the community and how the hospital can meet them. The board determines the scope of programs and services and the desired levels of quality and provides advice and counsel to the CEO in the implementation of plans and programs.

Questions for Discussion

1. Of the three summary job descriptions, which did you think was the best? Which did you think was the worst? Why?
2. Which description would provide the best guidance to a board that is struggling to focus its activities?
3. Are there components of all three job descriptions that have value? If so, what are they and why?

Board Chair Job Descriptions

For the same reasons that a written job description can help improve the board's performance, a job description for the board chairperson can help improve the leadership and overall effectiveness of the board. In fact, much of a board's effectiveness and development will depend upon the quality of its leadership. Unfortunately, one of the problems with many board leadership positions is a total lack of definition of what the chair is supposed to do. When this is the case, the effectiveness of the board often varies as board chairs change. Personality, rather than principle, dictates board function and focus.

Another common problem with the job of board chairperson is little or no formal orientation to or training for the job. That, of course, is directly related to the absence of a job description, which would form the basis for the orientation.

A significant benefit of a chair job description is that it enables the board to hold the person accountable for specific responsibilities and actions. The "it's not my job" defense, frequently used in delicate situations such as disciplining an errant board member, cannot be employed in the face of a job description that clearly defines the responsibility or action as part of the job. As with the board, the first step in constructing a job description for the chairperson is to delineate the responsibilities.

Exercise: Chairperson Responsibilities

Consider the following potential responsibilities of a board chair, then answer the questions that follow. The board chair

- keeps the mission of the organization foremost and articulates it as the basis for all board action
- understands and communicates the role and functions of the board, committees, medical staff, and management
- understands and communicates individual board member, board leader, and committee chair responsibilities and accountability
- acts as liaison between the board, management, and the medical staff
- plans agendas and meetings of the general board and executive committees
- presides over the meetings of the board and executive committee
- presides over or attends other board, medical staff, and other organization meetings
- enforces board and hospital bylaws, rules, and regulations (such as conflict-of-interest and confidentiality policies)
- appoints board committee chairs and members consistent with a systematic approach
- acts as a liaison between and among other boards in the health care system
- establishes board goals and objectives and translates them into annual work plans
- directs the committees of the board, ensuring that the committee works plans flow from and support the hospital and board goals, objectives, and work plans
- orientates new board members and arranges continuing education for the board
- ensures that effective board self-evaluation occurs
- builds cohesion among the leadership team of the board chair, CEO, and medical staff leader
- leads the CEO performance objective and evaluation process
- plans for board leadership succession

1. Of these board chairperson responsibilities, which do you think are most important? Why?

2. Are there any responsibilities that are not mentioned above that you believe are important? Identify them and add them to the list.

3. If you were to choose only five of the above responsibilities to form the basis of a job description for your board chairperson, which would you pick? Why?

4. Make sure that all the members of your board, or the members of the committee charged with drafting a job description for your board chair, answer question 3. Did they all choose the same five responsibilities? If yes, you have the basis of the board chairperson job description. If not, which responsibilities were chosen most frequently? This should form the basis of a board discussion as you develop a chairperson job description.

Trustee Job Descriptions

While some health care organizations have a job description for the board and perhaps even the chairperson, few have a job description for the individual board members. This is a major contributor to ineffective governance because many boards are composed of members who have very different ideas about what being a trustee means. In essence, these trustees each have implicit and wildly divergent job descriptions in their heads that cause them to act differently from one another and to regard the behavior of their colleagues as inappropriate.

Exercise: Developing Trustee Job Descriptions

Develop a list of possible trustee responsibilities. These might include

- attending all board and committee meetings
- reviewing all agenda materials in advance of the meetings
- completing new board member orientation
- keeping board deliberations confidential
- abiding by the vote of the majority
- communicating with the media and constituent groups

Once developed, rank the responsibilities from most important to least important. Have each trustee do this and compare the individual responses. From the comparison, develop a master list and ranking of individual board member responsibilities. This will then serve as both the foundation and bulk of the trustee job description.

Tips on Developing and Using Meaningful Board Job Descriptions

- Identify and prioritize the responsibilities and roles of the board. Translate these into a written job description of no more than three pages in length.
- Make certain that the board job description covers every aspect of the board's responsibilities and functions.
- Develop job descriptions for the chair and the individual member positions.
- Use the written job descriptions for the individual board member as the basis for developing performance criteria to determine reappointment to additional terms on the board.
- Use the chairperson job description to develop selection criteria and evaluate performance.
- Place the board job description, along with those of the chair and trustee, in each board agenda book.
- Routinely compare how the board is functioning with how the job description says it should function and note and discuss significant differences between the description and actual performance.
- Use the job description as a foundation for new trustee orientation and new board leadership training programs.
- As part of annual board self-evaluation, assess the appropriateness and value of the job descriptions. Refine or revise the job description as appropriate.

A Self-Assessment Questionnaire

The following brief survey can be used as a stand-alone survey or as part of an overall board self-evaluation process. Each board member should independently and anonymously rate the board's performance on the issues detailed in the following questions. The responses should be compiled, analyzed, and then discussed with the entire board present. The board should pay particular attention to those questions with significant variation in responses and those with predominately negative responses.

1. Does the board have a written job description for itself?

   ❑ Yes   ❑ No

   For individual board members?   ❑ Yes   ❑ No

   For the board chairperson?   ❑ Yes   ❑ No

2. The relative responsibilities, roles, and authority of the multiple boards in our corporate structure or health care system are spelled out in job descriptions for each board.

   ❑ Strongly Agree   ❑ Agree
   ❑ Somewhat Disagree   ❑ Disagree

3. The roles and responsibilities of our board are clearly defined in relation to those of the other boards within our health care system or organization.

   ❑ Strongly Agree   ❑ Agree
   ❑ Somewhat Disagree   ❑ Disagree

4. The board and CEO agree on their relative roles and responsibilities, and these are reflected in job descriptions for the board and CEO.

   ❑ Strongly Agree   ❑ Agree
   ❑ Somewhat Disagree   ❑ Disagree

5. Board and trustee job descriptions are shared with potential new board members as part of the trustee recruitment process.

   ❑ Strongly Agree   ❑ Agree
   ❑ Somewhat Disagree   ❑ Disagree

6. Board and trustee job descriptions are the basis for new board member orientation.

   ❑ Strongly Agree   ❑ Agree
   ❑ Somewhat Disagree   ❑ Disagree

7. Board job descriptions are reviewed as part of board leader training and development activities.

   ❑ Strongly Agree   ❑ Agree
   ❑ Somewhat Disagree   ❑ Disagree

8. Responsibilities of our board and individual members, as outlined in their job descriptions, are assessed as part of our board's ongoing self-evaluation process.

   ❑ Strongly Agree   ❑ Agree
   ❑ Somewhat Disagree   ❑ Disagree

9. The board annually reviews and revises its job description.

   ❑ Strongly Agree   ❑ Agree
   ❑ Somewhat Disagree   ❑ Disagree

Conclusion

Written job descriptions focus a board's efforts on performing the governance functions of a health care organization, as opposed to its managerial functions. Job descriptions for the board as a whole, for the chairperson, and for the individual board members clarify the rights and responsibilities of each and, in the ideal, resolve conflicts before they arise.

3

Orientation: Basic Building Blocks of Effective Boards

In the past, people invited to join a health care organization board would often protest that they knew nothing about health care or what a hospital or system board does. "Just come to the meetings and you'll pick it up pretty quickly," they were frequently told. Unfortunately, this "learn as you go," or "osmosis" approach to trustee orientation is still common today and, paradoxically, usually results in years of trustee disorientation. So this method is actually counterproductive to effective governance.

When hospitals were in a relatively unchallenged environment, characterized by predictability and stability, the contributions of, and the need for, a board were questionable. Boards did not contribute much (other than philanthropic giving) to the governance of their facilities. If effective boards were not necessary to hospitals, effective trustees were certainly not necessary to hospital boards. So there was little, if any, need for meaningful trustee orientation.

Now hospitals and other health care organizations exist in a challenging, changing, and turbulent environment, so it has become clearer that the board and the way it functions influences the viability of the hospital it governs. More specifically the board can affect the hospital in one of two broad ways: It can either be an asset or it can be a liability.

One characteristic of an effective board is the existence of a meaningful trustee orientation process that all new board members go through. Orientation should depend on more than luck, exhortations to read thick and boring manuals, individual initiative, and "osmosis." It should be a planned, deliberate process based partly on the board's stated functions, goals, and objectives and partly on the culture, values, and history of the entity.

Introduction to New Trustee Orientation

What is an effective orientation? It's more than simply a mechanism for providing new trustees with information. It's a structured process for beginning the complete development of the board member. While there is no specific orientation method that will work for all boards, effective orientation processes share a number of characteristics:

- understanding of the overall purpose of orientation
- clear distinction of the relative roles and responsibilities for orientation (in other words, who does what)
- clearly defined curriculum for the orientation process that directly relates to the hospital and board
- clearly defined mechanism and time frame for conducting the orientation
- ongoing evaluation of the orientation process that results in regular refinements and occasional revisions

What Is the Purpose of the Orientation Process?

If the purpose of the orientation process is not clear, it probably won't achieve much. Asking the purpose is likely to spark an obvious answer: to orient the new board member, of course. But orient the new trustee to what? Because many trustee orientations are not based on an answer to this explicit question, most are remarkably ineffective.

While each health care organization will determine its own purpose for trustee orientation, several broad purposes are common, including

- providing a general overview of the health care field to give new trustees a context in which the organization exists and functions

- outlining the culture, values, and norms of the organization and showing how the board recognizes and acts to perpetuate these key organizational characteristics
- providing a sense of the hospital's or system's history to help new trustees contribute to continuity in governance
- grounding new trustees in the organization's strategy as well as familiarizing them with the specific market characteristics that led to the development of the current strategic plan
- preparing new trustees for future board decisions and issues by reviewing local market trends
- providing new trustees with a solid picture of the hospital's finances
- reviewing recent, significant board decisions and their impact
- reviewing the structure, function, bylaws, and policies and procedures of the board, as well as its roles and responsibilities and those of any other boards within the organization
- providing an understanding of board values and culture and how they specifically affect the governance process
- reviewing the relationship of the organization to physicians and physician organizations as well as to other key constituency groups

Questions for Discussion

1. Which of the preceding purposes of orientation programs are the most important? Why?
2. Which of the purposes were achieved or addressed in your organization's trustee orientation process? Which were not?
3. How should your orientation process be modified to address any additional purposes you have identified?

Conducting Trustee Orientation

After the purposes of a new trustee orientation process are established, the next step is to determine who will conduct and oversee the process. This job often falls solely on the shoulders of the CEO. While it is appropriate for the CEO to be heavily involved in, and perhaps lead, the orientation process, remember that trustee orientation is a key component of board development. That's why the board should oversee the orientation process through a committee like the executive or board development committee.

A crucial component of the process is making newcomers feel comfortable with the board and the way it functions. Board members should also be involved in conducting key aspects of the process itself. Involvement of the board chair and several experienced trustees, as well as the chair of the committee to which the new trustee is likely to belong, is therefore desirable.

It is also appropriate to have outgoing trustees meet with newcomers to contribute a sense of continuity, or "passing the baton." In fact, by structuring the orientation process in order to coincide or conclude with a board retreat or board development session, the board as a whole can contribute to the orientation of new trustees.

One productive technique is for new trustees to attend a board self-evaluation session as soon as possible after they join the board. By participating in such a session, new trustees can see how the board examines and structures its function and how it evaluates its strengths and weaknesses. They'll also learn about board values and internal relationships among trustees and between the board and the CEO.

New trustees will be able to interact with other trustees outside the structure of board meetings, thereby building relationships, rapport, and board cohesiveness. Participation in a board self-evaluation session or retreat is an excellent way to accomplish what could otherwise take a year or more.

Besides retreats, other mechanisms for trustee orientation can include lectures, meetings, videotapes, written material, one-on-one discussions, tours of physical facilities, "auditing" various board committee meetings, and attendance at outside education programs.

One technique that many boards find particularly effective is pairing each new trustee with a seasoned trustee mentor. This approach not only gives new trustees specific resources for questions over time, but it can help provide a role model for new board members to observe effective governance in action. Furthermore, it signals to other trustees on the board that the mentors are those who have successfully mastered the techniques of good governance.

Questions for Discussion

1. Who conducts the trustee orientation in your facility? Why?
2. Who else could be involved in your orientation process to make it better?
3. Is the process overseen by the board as a whole or by a board committee, such as the board development, governance, or executive committee?
4. How long does a new trustee sit on your board before a retreat is held? Is this time frame appropriate?

Orientation Content

The next component of an effective trustee orientation process is a clearly defined curriculum. A meaningful orientation curriculum should be directly related to the mission and strategic direction of the health care organization and to board function and structure. But first the orientation process should provide a broad understanding of the health care field.

A number of issues should be reviewed to form this broad base:

- U.S. health care: its history, financing, and delivery and the reasons for, and impact of, the massive changes in the system; a review of payers and payment mechanisms, emphasizing the transition from fee-for-service to managed care and capitation
- hospitals and integrated delivery systems in general and within the context of the health care field
- the history and evolution of hospital and health care governance, including the legal authority and responsibilities of the board and its members and regulatory requirements
- physicians in the context of changes in health care, including the stress and pressures on doctors: loss of autonomy, reduced income, and increased scrutiny; the formation of

physician groups; and the relationship of physician groups to hospitals and purchasers
- the evolution of, and changes in, the medical staff, including its roles and responsibilities, and the changing relationship of the physician to the medical staff and of the medical staff to the hospital and board
- current health care trends and predicted future directions

Once this general orientation has been completed, conduct an orientation to the specifics of the organization and its governance. This orientation should review and discuss

- the history, mission, and values of the organization
- organizational structure, including a succinct review of hospital and medical staff bylaws
- hospital and system programs and services
- specific roles and responsibilities of the board, including a review of board policies and structure
- specific types of information (such as financial and quality reports) that will be routinely reported to the board and how to interpret this information
- hospital management roles, responsibilities, and structure
- medical staff roles, responsibilities, and structure
- the strategic plan and its current implementation status
- analysis of critical board relationships: boards of related corporations, subsidiaries, or parent
- review of board liability issues and protections

Once the orientation content is developed, determine the mechanisms and time frame for conducting the actual orientation: lectures, meetings, videotapes, written materials, retreats, one-on-one discussions, tours of physical facilities, "auditing" various board committee meetings, pairing each new trustee with a seasoned trustee mentor, and attendance at outside education programs.

In general, the more mechanisms used, the more effective the overall orientation process will be. Don't simply give new trustees a thick orientation manual and instruct them to "feel free to ask questions."

A meaningful orientation should not be a one-time event. Instead it should be constructed as an ongoing process over a period of several months, using various mechanisms and formats. But the process should not mark completion of the board's or new members' education. Ongoing education is a cornerstone of board development and effective governance, especially in today's turbulent climate. Activities that often are part of ongoing board education and development programs include

- attending regular leadership retreats
- devoting part of each board meeting to education on a specific topic
- sending board members to external educational programs
- subscribing to publications
- using audio- or videotapes designed for health care organization board members
- conducting periodic board self-assessments

Furthermore, just as the changing environment requires constant adjustment in the planning, structure, and operation of the health organization, it also requires continual change in the organization and operation of the governing board.

That's why the new trustee orientation process should be evaluated to make sure it is effective in preparing trustees for their demanding roles and modified as various changes in the health care field, the hospital, and the process of governance occur.

Questions for Discussion

1. Which of the broad health care issues and organization-specific information mentioned above are included in your orientation process?
2. What other issues are included? Should other issues be included?
3. How many of the learning formats and mechanisms mentioned in the previous section does your orientation program include? Which approaches do your board members find most effective?
4. When was your board's orientation process last evaluated or changed?

Tips for Effective Orientation Programs

- Make a point of involving board members in the new trustee orientation process.
- Charge a board committee to design, oversee, and periodically reevaluate the trustee orientation process.
- Ensure that the orientation process fulfills specific purposes or objectives and that these are regularly reviewed, modified as appropriate, and used to evaluate the overall effectiveness of the process.
- Ask new trustees to evaluate the orientation process after completing it. Also, ask trustees who have at least one to three years' experience on the board to think back to their own orientation process and suggest any additional topics that might have been helpful to new members. Then use this feedback in the overall trustee-orientation evaluation process.
- Schedule the trustee recruitment and orientation process to coincide with the annual board retreat so that a new board member can attend the retreat within the first three months of becoming a board member.
- Ensure that the orientation process offers pertinent information on the health care field in general and specific information on your health organization and its governance. In addition, ensure that the orientation process exposes new trustees to other board members and to leaders within the organization in ways that allow for socializing and building relationships.
- Use as many different mechanisms and formats as possible to convey information during the process.
- Support new trustee orientation with an ongoing program of board education and development.

A Self-Assessment Questionnaire

This brief survey addresses the board's roles and responsibilities in overseeing the orientation process. It can be used as a stand-alone survey or as part of an overall board self-evaluation.

Each trustee should independently and anonymously rate the board's performance on each of the following questions. Compile and analyze all the responses of the board and then discuss them with the entire board. Pay particular attention to questions that have significant variation in responses (where some trustees rate board performance high and some rate it low) and those questions with predominately negative responses.

1. Does the board have a formal new trustee orientation process?

   ❑ Yes   ❑ No

2. Are all new board members required to complete the process?

   ❑ Yes   ❑ No

3. Our new orientation process fulfills a specific purpose(s) or objective(s).

   ❑ Strongly Agree   ❑ Agree
   ❑ Disagree   ❑ Strongly Disagree

4. Our trustee orientation process provides information on broad health care issues and trends as well as information that is specific to our health care organization and its governance structure and function.

   ❑ Strongly Agree   ❑ Agree
   ❑ Disagree   ❑ Strongly Disagree

5. Several board members are involved in planning and conducting our process.

   ❑ Strongly Agree   ❑ Agree
   ❑ Disagree   ❑ Strongly Disagree

6. Our board orientation process includes opportunities to meet and socialize with other board members and organizational leaders.

   ❑ Strongly Agree   ❑ Agree
   ❑ Disagree   ❑ Strongly Disagree

7. The board, either as a whole or through one of its committees, is responsible for the design, conduct, and oversight of the process.

   ❑ Strongly Agree   ❑ Agree
   ❑ Disagree   ❑ Strongly Disagree

8. The board periodically evaluates the content, format, and process of board member orientation against the objectives it was designed to fulfill to ensure it continues to effectively meet its purpose(s).

❑ Strongly Agree   ❑ Agree
❑ Disagree   ❑ Strongly Disagree

9. The process is complemented and reinforced by board retreats and by an ongoing program of education and development.

❑ Strongly Agree   ❑ Agree
❑ Disagree   ❑ Strongly Disagree

10. Our current orientation process helps prepare new trustees to effectively lead our health care organization into the 21st century and to achieve our strategic goals.

❑ Strongly Agree   ❑ Agree
❑ Disagree   ❑ Strongly Disagree

11. The orientation process includes a component on the responsibility of the organization to its community and to the assessment and improvement of community health.

❑ Strongly Agree   ❑ Agree
❑ Disagree   ❑ Strongly Disagree

Conclusion

A meaningful new board member orientation process is a critical characteristic of effective governance. Just as a board will either help or hurt the organization it governs, so does a trustee either help or hurt the board to which he or she belongs. Successful boards and CEOs recognize this by constructing and conducting a formal and complete new trustee orientation process to get them off to the right start. They also regularly evaluate the process.

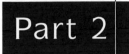

Part 2

Board Accountability

Assessing and Improving Your Community's Health

Healthy communities; community health assessment; improving the health status of communities; community accountability. These phrases, which are becoming increasingly familiar, reflect a changing dynamic in hospitals and health care organizations. As markets and other forces drive systemic reform, communities are becoming the focal point of change in health care.

With the growth of managed care and capitation, financial incentives for providers are shifting away from sickness care and toward prevention, wellness, and health maintenance. Under managed care and capitation, the incentives are clear for a health care organization to provide services that keep its enrolled population or covered lives healthy. But why should the board of the organization be concerned with the health status of its entire community, including those who are not enrolled in its health plans or among its covered lives?

Effective health care leaders realize that the overall community will inexorably influence the health of the organization's enrollees. Therefore, the health care organization must become intimately involved in and accountable for assessing and maximizing the health status of the entire community.

Health systems today are looking far beyond disease prevention and wellness to equally important issues, such as crime and poverty and their impact on overall community health. To be effective, health care leaders will have to measure their hospital's impact on community health and use the outcomes to improve the health status of the community. A community health improvement initiative is an effective investment in positioning for the future of managed care and fixed premium health care delivery. Perhaps more important, such an initiative is consistent with the missions of health care organizations and reflects an ethical commitment critical to the future of delivery.

It is easy to dismiss the focus on communities by conjuring up the American tradition of rugged individualism espoused by the 18th-century philosophy of John Locke and Thomas Hobbes. In essence, they encouraged a focus on the individual, with the belief that if the individual benefits first, the community will grow and benefit as a result. The American health care tradition of focusing on the treatment of sick individuals reflects this philosophy.

There is, however, another, and in fact older, American tradition that emphasizes the community. It is expressed in the writings of John Winthrop, the first governor of the Massachusetts Bay Colony, who in 1630 wrote, "We must delight in each other, make others' conditions our own, rejoice together, mourn together, labor and suffer together, always having before our eyes our community, as members of the same body."

What Is a Community?

The word "community" is frequently and often casually tossed around these days. Some hospitals have clearly defined communities, while larger integrated health delivery systems frequently have many disparate regions that make up their communities.

As hospitals merge and affiliate with other organizations, join larger integrated delivery systems, or even become part of national chains, the hospital's community becomes more diffuse and more difficult to define. A key question is, What is a community, and how is it defined?

Communities are like clouds. They can't be touched, only parts of them can be seen at one time from one perspective. They can change shape, form, and size in front of one's very eyes, and, depending on the economic or cultural winds, they can blow away. Even though communities often defy definition, a health care organization cannot begin to assess or improve the health status of its community until it can come up with some form of a working definition, including all of the community's demographic and economic subgroups.

Community Definition and Clarification: Questions for Discussion

Please consider and answer the following questions. This may be done by the individual trustee and then discussed with the board as a whole.

1. How does your organization primarily define its community now?
2. What are the other characteristics that your organization uses to define its community? Specify all of the following that apply: geographic area; economic diversity; age distribution; racial and ethnic populations; religious affiliations; particular disease categories (for example, cancer, tuberculosis, rehabilitation, psychiatry); and any other defining or limiting characteristics.
3. Can you develop a more specific or more encompassing definition of your community than the one you currently use?
4. Does the population of your community have any significant segments composed of identifiable categories of people (such as groupings by age, sex, race, education, income, or interest)?
5. How many of your board members are also members of your organization's defined community? Is that number or proportion appropriate?
6. How is your organization's community different today than it was five years ago?
7. How will your community likely be different five years from now?
8. What are the access points to health care in your community? (Do not limit your answer to only inpatient access points—think also of outpatient access points and those of prevention, education, screening, and others.)

Partnering for Community Health

No one organization can assume the responsibility for the health of an entire community. Why? Because community health is affected by a complex web of interconnected issues. These issues are broadly social, educational, and economic, and include but are not limited to such factors as substance abuse, crime, the stability and growth of the business environment, quality of education, religious institutions and affiliations, nutrition, the integrity of families, the stability or mobility of the population, teenage pregnancy, violence, recreation, and access to and quality of health care.

Because of the breadth and depth of these issues, it is impossible for a single organization to take complete responsibility for, and achieve meaningful results in, improving the health of its community. Community health is best addressed by a broad and deep network of partners. This partnership should reflect the complexity and diversity of the very issues that affect community health.

Thus, an effective partnership for community health will not only involve health care providers, but community and other organizations, such as churches, schools, and government agencies. This partnership should be a broad-based coalition that takes ownership of the development, articulation, and achievement of the vision of a healthier community.

It is important to understand that the hospital may not control or "own" the partnership. The purpose is not to aggrandize the hospital but to build many bridges to and improve the health of the community.

Therefore, participation in partnerships or coalitions to assess and improve community health requires health care leaders to have a big-picture systems view and a willingness to make the interests of the institution secondary to those of the community.

Partnerships for Community Health: Questions for Discussion

1. Which organizations are active in assessing and improving the health of your community?

2. With which of these organizations does your institution have a relationship or partnership?

3. Who are potential partners for your organization to collaborate with to improve the health of your community? (Think broadly; possible examples include other health care providers, foundations, churches, local school districts, state and local governments, businesses, community-based organizations, media, police and fire departments, and public health departments.)

4. How might your organization collaborate with such potential partners?

Tips for Effective Governance Involvement in Community Health

■ Define your community. Be specific in terms of geography, demographics, religious affiliations or groups, special categories (children's or women's hospital, for example).

■ Develop partnerships with other health care providers and community organizations that bring diverse resources together for community health assessment and improvement. Understand that the hospital may convene this partnership, but will not and should not dominate or control it.

■ Develop a shared vision, values, and plan with the partnership regarding community health, and specifically develop a broad definition of community health.

■ Using the definition of community health, develop a series of community health status indicators and routinely report them to both the partnership and your hospital board.

■ Using the health status indicators, develop annual community health status improvement goals and targets and measure performance and outcomes against these targets.

■ With the partnership, conduct routine assessments of the community's health status.

■ Consider creating a board committee that would oversee the organization's involvement in improving community health status and the community health partnership or coalition. Or, assign such a responsibility to an existing board committee.

■ Integrate existing initiatives for community health assessment and improvement with new ones; think in terms of creating and changing systems, not individual actions or initiatives.

- Hold your CEO accountable for community health through the CEO evaluation process: Develop specific CEO performance objectives based on community health status, education, and other indicators.
- Evaluate and, if necessary, revise the mission of the organization to ensure a commitment to community health.
- Build the concept of board responsibility for community health assessment and improvement into your board self-evaluation process.

The Causes of Death and Illness in the United States and Their Implications for Community Health Improvement

Almost half of all deaths in the United States are caused by behavioral factors such as smoking, the use of firearms, diet, and sedentary lifestyle. An article in the *Journal of the American Medical Association* of November 10, 1993, reported that in 1990 about 2,148,000 U.S. residents died.

Of these deaths 33.5 percent were due to heart disease; 23.5 percent were due to cancer; 6.7 percent were due to stroke or cerebrovascular disease; 4.3 percent were due to accidents; 4 percent were due to chronic obstructive pulmonary disease (emphysema); 3.7 percent were due to pneumonia and influenza; 2.2 percent were due to diabetes; 1.4 percent were due to suicide; 1.2 percent were due to chronic liver disease and cirrhosis; and 1.1 percent were due to AIDS.

The above factors are often referred as the "10 leading causes of death in the United States." The authors of the *JAMA* article point out that these are not really the root causes of deaths but rather the primary pathophysiological conditions at the time of death. The root causes are actually those external and genetic factors that bring about the conditions that precipitate death.

Using this logic, the authors identified a number of external contributors to death and quantified the approximate number of deaths actually caused by these factors. The most prominent external contributors to deaths and the estimated number of deaths caused by them in 1990 were

1. tobacco: 400,000 deaths, or 18.65 percent of the total number of deaths in 1990
2. diet and sedentary activity pattern: 300,000 deaths, or 13.9 percent
3. alcohol: 100,000 deaths, or 4.6 percent
4. microbial agents: 90,000 deaths, or 4.2 percent
5. toxic agents: 60,000 deaths, or 2.8 percent
6. firearms: 35,000 deaths, or 1.6 percent
7. sexual behavior: 30,000 deaths, or 1.4 percent
8. motor vehicles: 25,000 deaths, or 1.2 percent
9. illicit drug use: 20,000 deaths, or .9 percent

The authors also identify socioeconomic status and access to health care as important contributors to death, but they were unable to quantify the number of deaths these factors caused.

Almost half of all U.S. deaths in 1990 can be attributed to the factors identified above. This analysis should influence the actions of health care leaders and partnerships for community health improvement. For example, the way community health status is assessed by a health care organization should be broadened to include these contributory factors.

This analysis should also influence how society and health care organizations allocate their health care resources. The authors state that most health care dollars go to treat many of the conditions listed as the 10 most common causes of death, and only a very small fraction goes toward control of the many factors that actually cause death in this country and impose a substantial public health burden. Only about 5 percent of the total amount of money spent on health care in the United States annually is devoted to prevention.

Questions for Discussion

Please consider and answer the following questions. This may be done by the individual trustee and then discussed with the board as a whole.

1. What are the leading causes of morbidity and mortality in your community?

2. Was the answer to the above question generated by the results of a detailed community health assessment that was conducted by your organization in partnership with others? Was the answer based on factual information, regardless of source, or on assumption?
3. What percentage of your hospital's activities is currently devoted to illness and injury prevention as well as health maintenance? What percentage is devoted to treatment of illness and injury? Is this ratio appropriate? If not, how can it be changed?

Exercise: Factors Influencing Community Health

Following is a list of potential community health improvement initiatives. Each member of your board should independently and anonymously rank them in priority relative to their perceived value in meeting the needs of your community. Then tabulate, compare, and discuss the aggregate results. If your board could pick only five initiatives to implement, which would you pick and why?

- substance and alcohol abuse education and prevention
- teen pregnancy education and prevention
- infant mortality reduction
- adolescent health centers in schools
- neighborhood blood pressure watch
- glaucoma screening
- mallwalkers program
- violence prevention (gun buybacks, teaching conflict resolution and mediation skills, midnight sports leagues, and so forth)
- health fairs
- speakers' bureau
- child abuse prevention (parent modeling, education, surveillance, intervention, and other programs)
- fall prevention among the elderly
- automobile accident prevention
- childhood immunizations
- smoking cessation
- cardiovascular disease prevention

- mammography screenings
- radon testing
- water quality improvement
- Pap smear screening
- AIDS prevention programs (needle exchanges for drug users, sex education classes)
- physical fitness programs
- stress reduction programs
- stay-in-school programs
- food bank and food distribution activities
- neighborhood watch
- after-school activities
- Saturday night alcohol- and drug-free teen dances
- bicycle helmet giveaways, safety courses

What additional activities or initiatives to improve community health can you and your board identify?

A Self-Assessment Questionnaire

As indicated in the section "Tips for Effective Involvement in Community Health," boards can help hold themselves accountable for assessing and improving community health through their self-evaluation process. For boards who wish to do so, the issues covered in the following questionnaire may be of value.

This brief survey addresses the board's key roles and responsibilities in the oversight of community health. It can be used as a stand-alone survey or as part of an overall board self-evaluation process. Each trustee should independently and anonymously rate the board's performance on each of the following questions. Compile and analyze all the responses of the trustees and discuss them with the entire board. Pay particular attention to any questions that have significant variation in responses (where some trustees rate board performance high and some rate it low) and those with predominately negative responses. The discussion should result in the formation of a board action plan to increase the effectiveness of its oversight and improvement of the health of the communities served.

1. The mission of our organization reflects a strong commitment to the community and to the assessment and improvement of the health of the community.

   ❑ Yes   ❑ No

2. Our community is clearly defined.

   ❑ Yes   ❑ No

3. The board is an effective link between the hospital and the community.

   ❑ Strongly Agree   ❑ Agree
   ❑ Disagree   ❑ Strongly Disagree

4. Community organizations and leaders are regularly consulted about the value of the organization's services.

   ❑ Strongly Agree   ❑ Agree
   ❑ Disagree   ❑ Strongly Disagree

5. Board members are active spokespeople about health care issues in the community.

   ❑ Strongly Agree   ❑ Agree
   ❑ Disagree   ❑ Strongly Disagree

6. We regularly assess and can readily demonstrate that our organization provides a high level of benefit to our community.

   ❑ Strongly Agree   ❑ Agree
   ❑ Disagree   ❑ Strongly Disagree

7. The community benefit is regularly measured and quantified and exceeds in dollar value the amount of savings our organization annually realizes from our tax exemption.

   ❑ Strongly Agree   ❑ Agree
   ❑ Disagree   ❑ Strongly Disagree

8. There is a strong, trusting relationship between our organization and at least three community organizations in partnering to assess and improve the health of our communities.

   ❑ Strongly Agree   ❑ Agree
   ❑ Disagree   ❑ Strongly Disagree

9. We have a detailed plan with our partners to assess and improve the health of our community.

   ❏ Strongly Agree   ❏ Agree
   ❏ Disagree   ❏ Strongly Disagree

10. Our new board member orientation process includes a session on community health and the board's responsibility for it.

   ❏ Strongly Agree   ❏ Agree
   ❏ Disagree   ❏ Strongly Disagree

Conclusion

Improving community health involves much more than simply providing health care services, even to those populations that are underserved. It requires leadership commitment to and involvement with the community at all levels. More than that, it requires health care organization leaders to be willing to operate outside the traditional boundaries of the hospital, to reach beyond their defined patient populations or covered lives, to collaborate with nonproviders, and to seek and gain the trust of community leaders and organizations.

Perhaps most importantly, effectively improving community health requires health care organization leaders to be accountable to their communities and, ultimately, to themselves.

Board Oversight of Quality

Quality . . . you know what it is, yet you don't know what it is. But that's self-contradictory. But some things are better than others, that is they have more quality. But when you try to say what the quality is, apart from the things that have it, it all goes *poof!* There's nothing to talk about. But if you can't say what quality is, how do you know what it is, or how do you know that it even exists? If no one knows what it is, then for all practical purposes it doesn't exist at all. But for all practical purposes it really *does* exist. What else are grades based on? Why else would people pay fortunes for some things and throw others in the trash pile? Obviously some things are better than others. . . . But what's the "betterness"? . . . So round and round you go, spinning mental wheels and nowhere finding any place to get traction.
      What the hell is quality?

—*Robert M. Pirsig,* Zen and the Art of Motorcycle Maintenance

What Is Quality?

Just as quality in the events and objects of everyday life is difficult to pin down objectively, so is quality in health care. This will become increasingly apparent as the focus of health care shifts away from acute care toward community-based preventive care.
      Yet it's important to define quality for a very simple reason: If you can't define something, you can't measure it;

47

and if you can't measure something, you can't improve it consistently.

A good definition of quality can be found in the acronym RUMBA. That is, quality will be Realistic, Understandable, Measurable, Behavioral, and Achievable.

Now consider the following definitions of quality in health care:

Quality is doing the right things, the right way, the first time and every time.
—*Continuous quality improvement*

Quality is meeting or exceeding the expectations of our customers.
—*Several health care organizations*

[Quality is] a degree of excellence.
—*Merriam Webster's Collegiate Dictionary, 10th Edition*

Quality is conformance to norms.
—*Industrial definition*

The quality of a provider's medical care is the degree to which the process of care increases the probability of desired patient outcomes and reduces the probability of undesired outcomes, given the state of medical knowledge.
—*Congressional Office of Technology Assessment; Joint Commission on Accreditation of Healthcare Organizations*

Questions for Discussion

1. Which of the above definitions of quality meets the RUMBA test?
2. Which of the preceding definitions is most meaningful to your organization? Why?
3. Does your organization have a definition of quality? What is it? Where is it?
4. At the beginning of a board meeting, request that each trustee write the organization's definition of quality in his or her own words on a blank sheet of paper. Collect

the responses and collate and present them for discussion at the next meeting. Discuss the responses and compare them with the actual organizational definition of quality.

Toward Defining Quality

The first challenge for a board is to make certain that its organization has developed a working definition of quality that facilitates its measurement. But in addition to being measurable, it must also be meaningful. For example, in the preceding examples and questions, the most measurable definition of quality is achieving and maintaining accreditation; but is it the most meaningful? Many people would argue emphatically that it is not, that regulatory approval is no guarantee of true quality.

Perhaps the best way to conceptualize as well as define quality is to consider it from a variety of perspectives: medical, professional, and consumer. Patients' perspectives will probably be very different from their doctors'. Does this mean that only one of these two perspectives is valid?

Case Study

Consider this hypothetical situation: You are in a board meeting when, by chance, the board is presented with two quality-related reports. The first is from the chief of the medical staff, who reports on the results of a detailed and elegant six-month study of the quality of medical care in your growing outpatient surgery program. The study shows that, from a medical/clinical perspective, the quality of care in outpatient surgery is superb. Further, the study was examined by an outside researcher, who stated that its results are valid, reliable, and meaningful.

The very next report presented to the board is from the patient representative, who reports that outpatient surgery generates by far the largest numbers of patient complaints compared with any other area in the organization. Based on this, a six-month study of patient perceptions of quality in outpatient surgery was conducted. The results of the study clearly show that patients regard outpatient surgery quality of care as terrible, based on such criteria as waiting time and doctors' posttreatment instructions. This study has also been externally reviewed, and its results are also valid, reliable, and meaningful.

So exactly what is the quality of outpatient surgery care? Each trustee should consider this case study and compare and discuss his or her response.

How did you and your board answer the hypothetical question? Was the quality of care excellent or terrible? Or did you come up with another answer?

Another answer is, in fact, the right one: the care is both excellent from the medical/clinical perspective but terrible from the patients' perspective.

This answer strikes at the very heart of defining quality. The perspectives of quality that you and your board regard as being important will actually frame your practical definition. In the hypothetical situation, a board that included both the medical/clinical perspective and the patient perspective in its overall view of quality would have accepted and responded to both studies—rewarding and maintaining the excellent aspects and taking steps to improve the terrible.

The information that flows to a board about quality will be structured and influenced by its accepted quality perspectives. If a board chooses only one perspective, it will likely receive only information on that single, limited, and limiting aspect. If a board does not make explicit choices about which perspectives on quality it and the organization values, then its understanding of quality will be determined by the information it receives. This is a classic case of the tail wagging the dog.

Exercise: Perspectives on Quality

Please consider the different perspectives on quality listed below, and then answer the questions that follow.

- medical/clinical
- acute care outcomes
- patients' concerns
- community concerns

- measures of disease and injury prevention
- purchasers' of care concerns
- Joint Commission/government regulations
- cost/resource consumption
- media perspective
- healthy community measures
- malpractice insurance companies

Questions for Discussion

1. Which of the above perspectives on quality do you think are most important? Which are the least important? Why?
2. Which of the above perspectives are explicitly emphasized in your organization's definition of quality? Which are implicitly emphasized by your organization in its quality improvement efforts?
3. Are there other perspectives of quality that should be included?
4. Combine the board members' choices of the most important perspectives on quality into one list. Then, in discussion with the entire board, prioritize the perspectives. Once completed, consider the list: Your board has just constructed a rough definition of quality that can be assessed and measured by each specific perspective or component of quality.

Critical Success Factors

Effective health care organizations will have the following quality-related characteristics necessary for success:

- *Outcomes measurement and management:* The measurement and management of clinical and service outcomes, as well as inpatient and community-based outcomes, are critical to success under capitation.
- *Benchmarking:* This process involves identifying the best clinical and service practices from a quality and cost perspective and adopting these practices throughout the organization or system.
- *Total quality management and continuous quality improvement:* It's more productive to study the systems used to

provide clinical and service quality and correct flaws in those systems than it is to look for people's failures.

■ *Leadership at all levels:* Superb quality and service depends on strong and enlightened leadership at all levels of the organization. It also requires a long-term commitment from everybody, especially the board.

■ *Systems thinking:* This concept involves sharing values and assumptions, striving for the same vision, sharing the same view of the current environment, and applying these perspectives to maximize success for the entire system, not just one or some of its parts.

Questions for Discussion

1. Of the preceding characteristics, which do you think are most important to an organization's quality improvement efforts?
2. Which are present/absent in your organization? Which are most prominent?
3. Which type of board action could facilitate the development and improvement of the absent and least prominent characteristics?

Tips for Effective Board Oversight of Quality

■ Make certain your organization has developed a definition of quality, one that's broad enough to encompass community health, wellness, and prevention.

■ Make quality improvement a core organizational strategy, and closely link quality improvement activities to strategic priorities. For example, if a big push into ambulatory surgery is called for in the strategic plan, make certain that quality improvement in ambulatory surgery is emphasized in the plan, is funded by the budget, and is monitored by the board through a series of quality indicators.

■ Allocate sufficient financial resources to quality improvement (including information systems); for example, one to three percent of gross expense budget. Review annually the financial allocation to organizational or system quality as part of board oversight of budget.

- Provide a clear vision of the quality improvement process and its goals and reward compliance with the vision. Why is the organization or system doing this—to be the best it can be or simply to satisfy regulatory and accrediting requirements?
- Prepare information about the quality and performance of your organization for key stakeholder groups, such as the community, media, purchasers, and other health care providers.
- Oversee the systemwide quality improvement process; don't focus only on the inpatient, acute care side. Recognize that as health care moves into the community, the definition and measurement of quality will also move there.
- Focus on systems improvement and integration, not individuals.
- Ensure that lessons learned from quality improvement efforts are disseminated and adopted throughout the organization.
- Develop specific CEO performance objectives based on measurable and achievable quality goals, and hold your CEO accountable for quality through the performance-evaluation process.
- Lead by example; initiate quality improvement in governance and medical staff leadership processes.

Economics of Prevention

As the focus of health care shifts from inpatients and sickness to community-based prevention and wellness, the issue of defining and measuring quality changes with it. Many health care organizations are placing a greater emphasis on prevention and wellness than ever before. However, Office of Technology Assessment (OTA) studies ("The Price of Prevention," *Scientific American,* April 1995) have found that few preventive services pay for themselves and, in some cases, cost more than treating the disease. So boards must compare the effectiveness against the cost of preventive services to weed out those that promise more than they deliver.

Primary prevention, such as immunization and counseling, directly changes the likelihood that someone will develop a disease or injury and tends to be cost-effective. Secondary prevention, such as screening tests, have no such effect, according to the OTA studies.

The following are some examples of cost-effective primary preventive services:

- prenatal care for poor women (every dollar spent saves from $1.70 to $3.38)
- childhood immunizations
- prospective testing for congenital disorders

Questions for Discussion

1. What percentage of your organization's budget is devoted to prevention, as opposed to treatment?
2. Of your organization's preventive activities, what percentage are primary prevention, and what percentage are secondary prevention?
3. What are some examples of your preventive activities?
4. Are your prevention activities based on the results of a community health assessment?

Exercise: Board Indicators of Quality

There is no single measure that will provide a meaningful overall picture of quality. Rather, quality represents a combination of variables and indicators.

The following are some potential quality indicators:

- mortality rates
- childhood immunization rate in the community
- cholesterol screening
- nosocomial infection rates
- mammography screening
- adverse drug reactions or interactions
- rate of Pap smears for cervical cancer
- tobacco use rates
- success rates for smoking cessation programs
- returns to the emergency department within 72 hours of treatment

- drug abuse rates
- drug prevention and counseling programs use and success rate
- unplanned returns to surgery
- obesity rates in the community
- success rates for nutrition and exercise programs
- rate of prenatal care for women in the first trimester of pregnancy
- percentage of community members between the ages of 23 and 40 who have seen a physician or other provider in the previous two years
- number and percentage of primary care physicians accepting new patients
- medication error rates
- patient complaints

Questions for Discussion

1. Which of the preceding quality indicators does your board currently receive information about?
2. If your board could receive only five of the quality indicators routinely, which ones would you choose? Why?
3. Of all the quality indicators that your board receives, what percentage relates to inpatient acute care? What percentage relates to outpatient acute care? What percentage relates to community health? What percentage relates to nonacute outpatient care? Why is this the case?

A Self-Assessment Questionnaire

The following brief survey addresses the board's key roles and responsibilities in the oversight of quality. It can be used as a stand-alone survey or as part of an overall board self-evaluation process.

Each trustee should independently and anonymously rate the board's performance on each of the following questions. Compile and analyze all the responses of the board and discuss them with the entire board. Pay particular attention to questions with significant variation in responses and those with predominately negative responses.

1. Quality is an agenda item at every board meeting.

   ❑ Strongly Agree   ❑ Agree
   ❑ Somewhat Disagree   ❑ Disagree

2. The information the board receives about the quality of care and the quality improvement program is complete and adequate for board-level discussion and decision making.

   ❑ Strongly Agree   ❑ Agree
   ❑ Somewhat Disagree   ❑ Disagree

3. The board routinely receives quality indicators.

   ❑ Strongly Agree   ❑ Agree
   ❑ Somewhat Disagree   ❑ Disagree

4. The quality indicators are not limited only to acute, inpatient care, but also include indicators of quality in outpatient settings and community health.

   ❑ Strongly Agree   ❑ Agree
   ❑ Somewhat Disagree   ❑ Disagree

5. The real purpose of our quality improvement activities is to gain and maintain accreditation.

   ❑ Strongly Agree   ❑ Agree
   ❑ Somewhat Disagree   ❑ Disagree

6. We have valid empirical data that demonstrate the quality of care our organization provides.

   ❑ Strongly Agree   ❑ Agree
   ❑ Somewhat Disagree   ❑ Disagree

7. We provide information to our community about the quality of our care.

   ❑ Strongly Agree   ❑ Agree
   ❑ Somewhat Disagree   ❑ Disagree

8. We have a meaningful, measurable definition of quality.

   ❑ Strongly Agree   ❑ Agree
   ❑ Somewhat Disagree   ❑ Disagree

9. Our board spends the same amount of time and energy overseeing quality as we do finance.

   ❏ Strongly Agree   ❏ Agree
   ❏ Somewhat Disagree   ❏ Disagree

10. Our organization provides high-quality care.

   ❏ Strongly Agree   ❏ Agree
   ❏ Somewhat Disagree   ❏ Disagree

Conclusion

The quality of care that your organization provides begins and ends with your board. Effective board involvement in and oversight of quality hinges on two critical components: meaningful commitment to quality and meaningful information about quality. As the nature of health care, and therefore quality, moves to the community arena, board attention and commitment must lead this transformation.

Self-Evaluation: Mark of Good Governance

The unexamined life is not worth living.

—*Socrates*

No one ever knows us quite as well as we know ourselves.

—*Sigmund Freud*

All governing boards are familiar with the evaluation of performance. Boards evaluate the performance of the CEO, the medical staff, the financial operations of the organization, the progress made toward improving the health of the community, and many other areas. In fact, most boards are very comfortable evaluating performance—unless, of course, it's their own performance that is being evaluated.

Self-evaluation—the board's assessment of its own performance, structure, and function—is perhaps the board's most important education and development activity. Although a relatively new concept in the fields of corporate governance, many health care organization boards have long engaged in regular self-evaluation in order to identify their strengths and weaknesses and improve their overall performance.

Board self-evaluation has been defined as "an organized process by which the board regularly reexamines its goals and objectives, structure, processes, and collective and individual performance, and then reaffirms its commitment by adopting new goals and improved methods of operation."[1]

Fundamentals of Board Self-Evaluation

There are two basic reasons why health care system and hospital boards should perform periodic self-evaluations. The first is that today's unforgiving health care environment demands nothing less than excellence in governance. The second is that a well-constructed self-evaluation process can help a board improve its performance and achieve and maintain excellence in governance.

The process provides a board with a structured opportunity to both look back and to plan ahead. The process enables the board to ask itself such questions as

- What are we doing well?
- What could we be doing better?
- What are our objectives?
- How well did we achieve our objectives?
- Why didn't we achieve our objectives?

The board then uses the answers to the questions to develop an action plan to improve its performance and establish new goals.

Most self-evaluations use questionnaires or surveys. Questions are typically structured in one of two ways: close- and open-ended. Close-ended questions, which are used most often, ask respondents to select their answers from specific options, such as yes and no or a range of possible responses along a given scale. Open-ended questions enable respondents to provide their own thoughts or opinions in narrative form.

The advantage to close-ended questionnaires is that they can be answered more quickly and, therefore, can help

---

1. Richard Umbdenstock, Winnifred Hageman, and Barry Bader, *Improving and Evaluating Board Performance* (Rockville, Md.: Bader & Associates, 1986).

boost the overall level of survey response from the board. Open-ended surveys usually take more time to complete but allow board members to amplify and clarify their thoughts and opinions on specific issues. Questionnaires often include both types of questions.

Here are some examples of each type of question:

Close-Ended

1. Does your organization have a formal mission statement?

   ❏ Yes   ❏ No   ❏ Don't know

2. Is your organization achieving its mission? (circle one)
   a. Yes, completely
   b. Yes, primarily
   c. Yes, partially
   d. No, not the most important part
   e. No, not at all
   f. Don't know

3. To what degree does the performance of the board influence achievement of the organization's mission? (circle one)

   Completely   Somewhat   Not at all
   1   2   3   4   5

Open-Ended

4. Briefly describe your understanding of your organization's mission (25 words or fewer).

5. Briefly write down your understanding of the three primary roles and responsibilities of the board.

Once the self-evaluation survey format is developed, each trustee is given a questionnaire to complete independently and confidentially. Each trustee then returns the completed questionnaire to a designated facilitator or consultant via mail or fax.

All of the responses are then compiled into one question-naire, which allows analysis of the aggregate results. The responses of the board and the analysis are subsequently used to facilitate discussion among board members. This facilitated discussion is the real meat of the process.

Other methods can be used to generate facilitated discussion among a board over its strengths and weaknesses. These include computer-based polling technologies, which enable a board to respond to questions in real time with the aid of separate keypads and a master computer. The computer instantly tabulates responses and displays them graphically for the board to discuss. Using this approach, a board can develop questions and poll itself anonymously during a self-evaluation retreat.

Another, less structured approach involves a facilitator simply stimulating an open-ended discussion among a board on strengths, weaknesses, and opportunities for improvement. The facilitator then probes and challenges the board in a spontaneous manner until the most significant governance issues are identified and examined.

In each of the three approaches, facilitated discussion of board performance is key. From the facilitated discussion a number of issues, questions, and concerns will arise. These form the basis for developing a board action plan. The plan lists those areas to be addressed and strengthened by the board, prioritizes the issues to be addressed, establishes deadlines, and assigns responsibility for action. For example, action items may be assigned to a standing board committee, an ad hoc committee, the whole board, management, or the board chairman and the CEO, to name a few.

Often, several items on the action plan can be addressed during the board retreat itself (such as the creation or elimination of board committees and the agreement to establish or modify term limits). The action plan is key to improving the performance of the board. The development of the action plan and strategies for its implementation typically marks the end of the facilitated board self-assessment discussion.

It is important to stress that simply discussing a board's performance and developing an action plan do not constitute a successful self-evaluation. An action plan must not only be developed to improve board performance, it also must be implemented. It is up to the board and CEO to implement the action plan once the self-evaluation session is over. Unfortunately, many boards never implement the action plans that were developed.

For these boards, the self-evaluation exercise is a waste of time. It does not improve board performance and actually hinders it by causing frustration among the board members.

Questions for Discussion

1. Which one of the three approaches to conducting a board self-evaluation did your board use? Which was most effective? If your board did not conduct a self-evaluation, which approach is most appealing?
2. If your board has conducted self-evaluations in the past, did they result in the development of an action plan to improve board performance or structure? How many and which of the items on the action plan were successfully implemented by the board?
3. Why were some board improvement action plan items successfully implemented and some not?
4. What were the most challenging aspects of participating in a board self-evaluation? What were the most rewarding aspects?
5. What five strategies or actions would improve the structure, function, or decision-making process of your board?

Better Self-Evaluations through the Use of Annual Goals and Objectives

Most health care organizations have annual organizational goals and objectives that are part of, or flow from, the strategic plan. These organizational objectives usually form the basis for the CEO performance objectives and evaluation. These same organizational objectives should also form the basis for annual board goals and objectives.

The development of objectives for both the CEO and the board facilitates coordination and teamwork among members of the organization's leadership team. Most boards understand the need for CEO performance objectives, even though they don't actually develop them. But few understand the need for annual board goals and objectives.

When boards are asked during retreats whether they performed well during the past year the response is usually a resounding "Yes, we did a good job." When asked whether the board had annual goals or objectives against which to measure their performance, the response is almost always "No." In effect, these boards are saying, "We don't know what our job is, but we did it very well!" When confronted with this restatement of their logic, most boards realize the value of annual board goals and objectives.

Just as the CEO performance objectives focus on the work, time, and attention of the CEO, so do annual board goals and objectives focus on the work and structure of the board. Without them, a board might be tempted to think and act as if its work, meetings, and decisions are routine—the same from year to year. That mindset is in fact why some boards regress into a stultifying sameness of function. Even when there is environmental upheaval, the board does not perceive the need to modify its focus or function.

Entrenched in the fear that usually accompanies change, this complacency is the antithesis of good governance. It's almost as if the board has been preserved in amber.

Consideration of specific board goals and objectives reveals one of the key characteristics of effective governance: a dynamic, evolving board function and form. Yet the only disciplined way for a board to adopt this flexibility is to do so in the context of structured goals and objectives that are explicitly developed on a regular basis.

These goals and objectives should reflect organizational goals and changes in the organization's focus and environment. They also help the board to understand its overall roles and responsibilities and improve its ability to govern.

These two types of board goals and objectives—those that focus the board on supporting achievement of the organization's strategic plan and those that help the board improve its own ability to govern—form the basis for the self-evaluation. The board assesses its performance relative to the accomplishment of specific board goals, not relative to vague notions about what the board should have done or should be doing.

A practical way to enhance leadership effectiveness is to develop the annual CEO performance objectives and the annual board objectives at the same time. Further, the board and CEO should have input into both sets of objectives. This creates a formal "expectations exchange," in which, through mutual discussion and negotiation, the board clarifies its expectations of the CEO, and the CEO clarifies his or her expectations of the board.

Once this clarification is accomplished, the practical distinction between governance and management has been established and the foundation for effective leadership for the coming year has been laid. Further, the board self-evaluation process will now be based on specific objectives and will likely be more effective in improving future board performance.

Questions for Discussion

1. Does your board develop annual board goals and objectives? Do these goals and objectives include both those that support achievement of the organization's strategic plan and those that help the board better understand its overall roles and responsibilities and improve its ability to govern? How successful has your board been in accomplishing its goals?
2. If your board develops annual board goals and objectives, are they routinely used as the basis for its self-evaluation?
3. If your board does not develop annual goals and objectives for itself, look back over the past year and list the implicit board goals and objectives (those areas of greatest board attention and focus). Were these areas of board focus consistent with the organizational strategy? Did they help the board lead the organization in new directions, or did they reinforce the past?
4. What are the three most important board goals and objectives for the coming year? How does your answer compare with those submitted by your fellow board members?

Tips on Effective Board Self-Evaluation

- Never conduct the board self-evaluation session as part of a regular board meeting.
- Use an outside facilitator, who can provide focus, structure, and an objective perspective for the self-evaluation session. When the CEO, board chairman, or other internal person tries to facilitate a board retreat, problems due to lack of objectivity, hidden agendas, personality conflicts, and many other issues frequently result.
- Develop annual board goals and objectives and use them as the basis for the self-evaluation questionnaire and the facilitated discussion session.
- Make certain that only board members, and perhaps one or two other people who regularly attend board meetings, are invited, complete the self-evaluation questionnaire, and participate in the self-evaluation retreat. Having non-board members attend what is supposed to be a board self-evaluation will inhibit or sidetrack meaningful discussion.
- Tailor the self-evaluation to address the specific needs and goals of each board. Work with the facilitator before the retreat to familiarize him or her with the specific characteristics of the hospital and board.
- Don't hold the self-evaluation session at the usual board meeting location. A new environment helps create a more relaxed atmosphere, which is conducive to free discussion and effective group process.
- Make certain that the self-evaluation results in the development of a board action plan. This plan should prioritize the strategies and steps to improve board structure, function, or process. It should assign responsibility for investigation or implementation of the action items and establish deadlines for completion as well.
- If the self-evaluation is conducted as part of a broader governance retreat, allow at least three hours for the entire process (review and discussion of the questionnaire results, discussion of other issues, and development and prioritization of the action plan).
- Be flexible. Don't make your agenda too rigid, but don't have a completely free and loose "anything goes" agenda either. If the self-evaluation discussion veers into

unanticipated areas, instruct your facilitator to explore the area and to facilitate the development of action plan items relative to it.

- Be honest during the facilitated self-evaluation discussion. If there are aspects of a board function that you are concerned about, or if you have suggestions that would improve board function or structure, express them. Focus your comments on principles, not on personalities.

Areas for Board Self-Evaluation

When a board conducts a self-evaluation, the members must focus on the many governance areas they wish to evaluate in addition to the accomplishment of previously established board goals and objectives.

Consider the following areas related to effective governance that can be addressed during a self-evaluation:

- mission stewardship
- board structure and organization
  —board size
  —number of boards in a system
  —number of board committees
  —board policies and procedures
- strategic planning
- quality improvement
- medical staff credentialing
- finance
- community health and relations
- board education and development
  —new trustee identification, selection, and orientation
  —continuing board education
  —board retreats
- board function
  —board meeting frequency and length
  —agenda development and relevance
  —effectiveness of governance information
  —quality of board meetings and discussion
  —quality and timeliness of the board's decision-making process

- board relationships
  - —board-CEO relationship
  - —board-medical staff or other physician group relationships
  - —board relationship with its members and committees
  - —board relationship with other boards affiliated with the organization
- board leadership
- succession planning for board leadership, including the board chair and the board committee chairs
- board conflict-of-interest and confidentiality policies
- mechanisms for removing nonperforming board members from the board

Questions for Discussion

1. Which areas of board assessment are most critical for your board to address? Why?
2. In which areas does your board perform most effectively? Why?
3. What other areas of governance should your board address during its self-evaluation process?

Conclusion

Routine and meaningful self-evaluations that result in specific actions to improve board structure, function, and overall performance are crucial means of promoting excellence in governance. They are also an important way for a board to demonstrate participation in, and support for, the organization's commitment to continuous improvement. Boards that only infrequently step back to engage in self-assessment miss key opportunities to develop a shared understanding of roles and responsibilities, a common vision, and a renewed commitment to governance.

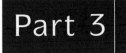

Part 3

Strategic Planning and Information

Developing a Community-Focused Mission

A man comes before your board with a briefcase full of magic pills, offering to sell them for 15 cents each. If people took the pill, they would never again experience illness or injury, and existing disease would be cured. Your board is asked if it wishes to buy the pills and give one to each person in the community.

Think about this hypothetical situation for a moment. If your board distributes the pills to the community, the institution could well go out of business. If the board buys the pills and destroys them, or charges an exorbitant sum for them, the institution would profit and continue to exist, but would do so at the expense of the community. What should the trustees do in this situation? What should guide them in making the decision? The answer to both questions should be found in the mission of the organization.

As health care changes, the character and function of governance will also change. For example, governance of integrated delivery systems (IDSs) may be very different from governance of hospitals; the governance of a facility is very different from the governance of an organization that is responsible for the health of a community. Yet one of the constants of governance is the accountability of the board to the mission of the organization it governs.

Effective governance requires an effective mission. Why? In tough and turbulent times, a board without a clear sense of its organization's purpose is likely to focus on short-term issues, overreact to events, and contribute to organizational drift and disarray. Further, the board is more likely to focus on finances rather than on the external community and constituents.

What Is a Mission?

The mission is the primary force that holds an organization together. Thus, validity of the mission and the degree to which the organization is successful in achieving it must be the board's central concern. Effective governance requires an effective mission. But what is an effective mission?

Here are two compelling definitions of the mission and its importance:

> The mission statement is the job description of your hospital stated in community terms. . . . The statement is a tool designed to communicate what the hospital stands for. It is the beginning point of discipline that will allow you to sensibly appraise requests for money, new equipment, new staff, and new facilities. The mission statement is the beginning (and end) of your plan.
> —*Norman H. McMillan,* Planning for Survival

> The mission focuses the organization on action. It defines the specific strategies needed to attain the crucial goals. It creates a disciplined organization. It alone can prevent the most common degenerative disease of organizations . . . splintering their always limited resources.
> —*Peter Drucker, "What Business Can Learn From Non-Profits,"* Harvard Business Review, *July–August 1989*

A mission defines what your organization is and what it is not. A key characteristic of a good mission is that it helps the board make difficult decisions by giving the trustees a guiding set of principles.

A mission should be current, relevant, and specific enough to position the hospital or health care organization uniquely within its service area. To help ensure that the mission clearly and precisely states your hospital's reason for being, it should identify the purpose, philosophy, and perhaps the values of the organization and should include a focus on the health needs of the community. A mission can have the following components:

- type of organization: teaching, government, religious
- scope of services: long term, acute, continuum of care, exclusions (if any)
- service area/intended customers: city, county, region, particular demographic group (women, children, or cancer or tuberculosis patients, for example)
- type or dimensions of care: spiritual, psychological
- strengths, limitations: cost, access, quality, special affiliations
- community focus

According to the Endowment Leadership Program of the Eli Lilly Foundation, an effective board has a collective answer to the following three questions:

1. What do we believe?
2. Whom do we serve?
3. What do we do?

The first two questions should be answered in the mission; the third question flows from the mission. Thus, an effective mission provides the basis for a board to answer these questions.

Mission Case Examples

Following are four sample mission statements for your review. Please evaluate them in relation to one another using the questions that follow.

Mission 1: The mission of General Hospital is to provide quality, cost-effective health care services to the people of Blue County and our regional service area.

Mission 2: Regional Medical Center will ensure the highest quality services to our patients, guests, and physicians while achieving a balance between community needs and available resources, thus sustaining a viable financial position. We will provide referral services to residents of surrounding areas where market or internal needs exist, or where RMC can attain a distinct competitive position.

Our Values

- *Commitment:* Our foremost commitment is to provide the highest quality services to our patients, guests, and physicians in fulfillment of our mission.
- *Compassion:* We will show compassion for those in need, providing for the young and the old, the rich and the poor, regardless of race and creed. We will return to our community the investment of trust placed in us, through quality care, education, and participation in local activities.
- *Communications:* Our communications will be open and honest in our dealings with patients, employees, physicians, and the community.
- *Competence:* We will value competence in the abilities of our employees and volunteers to serve those entrusted to our care. The achievement of excellence will be recognized and rewarded.

Mission 3: Good Works Hospital, as a Catholic community organization, is committed to

- offering a full range of services usually provided by a community hospital to the residents, businesses, and communities of Rural Valley
- offering specialized services in trauma, neonatology, perinatology, intensive care, coronary care, orthopedics, oncology, and rehabilitation
- maintaining and assisting a competent medical staff to provide quality medical care
- retaining a qualified nursing staff and hospital support staff in order to maintain a high standard of hospital care
- offering a work environment which enhances and recognizes excellence and creativity among employees and volunteers

- identifying and developing outpatient services and health education programs to meet the specific needs of the hospital service area
- providing current technology, facilities, and equipment
- managing the hospital's finances in a prudent, responsible manner in order to meet the present and future needs of the hospital
- addressing the future health care needs of the service area through continual analysis of trends, refinement of existing services, and introduction of new services

Mission 4: The mission of Valley Community Hospital is to make the community of Clover County the healthiest place to live in America by the year 2000.

Questions for Discussion

Using the description of what should be in a mission statement in the "What Is a Mission" section, consider the following questions. This should be done individually by each trustee and then discussed with the board as a whole.

1. What components of a good mission statement does each example include?
2. What components of a good mission statement are excluded from each?
3. Which mission statement creates the most unique identity for the hospital?
4. Which mission example would provide the best guidance to a board confronting a difficult decision (such as merger, closure, offering, or curtailment of specific services)?
5. Of the four mission examples, which one do you like best? Why?

Exercises: Mission Development and Improvement

The following exercises are intended to help your board develop a mission for your organization or improve an existing mission.

Exercise 1

Please consider the following quote from *The Autobiography of Mohandas K. Gandhi* and the questions that follow it.

It is my firm conviction that it is not good to run public institutions on permanent funds. A permanent fund carries in itself the seed of the moral fall of the institution. . . . When such an institution ceases to have public support, it forfeits its right to exist. Institutions maintained on permanent funds are often found to ignore public opinion, and are frequently responsible for acts contrary to it. The trustees have become the owners and are responsible to none. I have no doubt that the ideal is for public institutions to live, like nature, from day to day. The institution that fails to win public support has no right to exist as such. The subscriptions that an institution annually receives are a test of its popularity and the honesty of its management: I am of the opinion that every institution should submit to that test.

1. Does Gandhi's view of "public institutions" have any applicability for your hospital or health care organization?
2. To whom are the trustees of your organization responsible?
3. In a "new reality" or redesigned health care environment, what "tests" should your organization have to pass in order to survive?

Exercise 2

At the beginning of a board meeting, and without prior notice, request that each trustee write the hospital mission in his or her own words on a sheet of paper. This should be done in 50 words or less and in no more than five minutes. Have the responses collected, collated, and presented for discussion at the next board meeting. An effective board with an effective mission will demonstrate a very consistent response. Be alert for inconsistent responses and for responses that demonstrate divisions within the board. Discuss the responses of the board, then compare them to the actual mission.

Exercise 3

Consider and discuss with the board the following:

1. What would be the impact on your mission if your organization lost its tax-exempt status?
2. Would your mission in any way change if universal coverage is enacted? How?

3. Does your mission provide guidance regarding the evaluation of potential mergers, affiliations, or formations of IDSs?
4. Does your mission focus on the institution or on the community?

Tips for an Effective Governance Focus on Mission

- Clarify and articulate the mission, vision, goals, and strategic plan and make them the foundation for board decisions
- Place the mission statement on the first page of every board
  agenda book and every board committee agenda book. (This
  is useful for the medical executive committee as well.)
- Track board decisions for consistency and relevance to the
  mission; provide an annual written update on results of past
  board decisions and their impact on mission fulfillment.
- Make education regarding the mission and the board's role
  in mission stewardship the foundation of the new trustee
  orientation program and the leadership training program
  for new board leaders.
- Reevaluate the mission annually with the entire board and
  explicitly decide to either reaffirm it or revise it.
- Develop annual board objectives and an annual board
  work plan that flow from and support the mission and
  strategic plan.
- Prominently include the role of the board and the individual trustee in mission oversight in a written, clearly
  defined statement of board roles and responsibilities.
  Develop a written job description for the board and for the
  individual trustee.
- Construct and evaluate board meeting agendas with mission relevance as the prime criterion.
- Clarify the roles and functions of the board committees.
  Develop annual committee work plans that flow from and
  support the mission.
- Integrate a mission stewardship and fulfillment component
  into a board self-evaluations and use the results to change,
  fine-tune, and improve board function and structure.
- Hold the CEO accountable for mission fulfillment through
  the CEO evaluation process; develop specific CEO performance objectives based on mission fulfillment.

Mission Stewardship and Mission Revision

To be an effective steward of the mission, the board must be involved in

- the development of the mission
- the articulation of the mission
- ongoing monitoring of the mission and its continued relevance
- revision of the mission when appropriate

With all of the dizzying changes in health care and hospitals, it is an appropriate time for most boards to ask: Is our mission still relevant?

Many well-known organizations have examined and revised their missions, and in doing so have changed their identities and continued to exist with a new focus. Following are several examples:

March of Dimes

Original mission: The elimination of polio
Revised mission: Combating arthritis and birth defects

American Red Cross

Original mission: To "hold itself in readiness in the event of war or any calamity . . . considered national"
Revised mission: The preservation and improvement of public health

Dartmouth College

Original mission: To educate and Christianize the Indians of New England
Revised mission: A general liberal arts college

These examples indicate that many different situations can precipitate a revision of an organization's mission. These include

- fulfillment of the original mission
- a change in market conditions, such as the emergence of unmet needs or unnecessary and wasteful duplication of services

- new industry trends
- systemic restructuring of financial and/or delivery systems
- new legislative requirements or initiatives

Many of these situations are present or likely to emerge in the near future. Thus, many health care organizations may need a revised mission in order to remain relevant and viable in a changing environment.

Health care is moving away from individual care of the acutely sick and toward maintaining the health of a community; from hospitals to IDSs; from fragmented care with an acute care focus to a continuum of care with an outpatient focus.

Do these and other trends suggest that an examination of your mission for possible revision is appropriate? If so, consider moving the mission away from an internal hospital focus and toward an external community focus.

Mission Evaluation and Review: Questions for Discussion

1. What are the key health care issues facing your community?
2. Is the organization your current mission statement describes best positioned to deal with the health care needs of your community today and tomorrow?
3. Are major activities and programs your hospital is now engaged in relevant to the achievement of its mission? If not, what does the dissonance say about what your organization ought to be focused on?
4. Does your mission address strategic partnerships or alliances that indicate your hospital's linkage with others in the community to meet the health care needs of the population?
5. What do you think health care delivery will look like in your community 5 to 10 years from now? Does your mission statement describe an organization that is likely to play a key role in your community's health care future?

The Board's Role in Mission: A Self-Assessment Questionnaire

The following brief survey addresses the board's key roles and responsibilities in mission oversight. It can be used as a stand-alone survey, or it may be used as part of an overall board self-evaluation process.

Have each trustee independently and anonymously rate the board's performance using each of the following questions. Compile and analyze all the responses of the board and discuss them with the entire board. Pay particular attention to questions with significant variation in responses (where some trustees rate board performance high and some rate it low) and those with predominately negative responses. The discussion should result in the formation of a board action plan to improve its mission oversight.

1. Has our board approved a written statement of the mission of our hospital or health care organization?

   ❏ Yes   ❏ No

2. The board is knowledgeable about and supportive of the principles of our hospital mission.

   ❏ Strongly Agree   ❏ Agree
   ❏ Disagree   ❏ Strongly Disagree

3. The board provides direction for implementing our mission, including guidelines and criteria.

   ❏ Strongly Agree   ❏ Agree
   ❏ Disagree   ❏ Strongly Disagree

4. The board reviews proposals for programs and services to ensure they are consistent with the mission.

   ❏ Strongly Agree   ❏ Agree
   ❏ Disagree   ❏ Strongly Disagree

5. The board monitors the organization's programs and activities to ensure they are consistent with the mission.

   ❏ Strongly Agree   ❏ Agree
   ❏ Disagree   ❏ Strongly Disagree

6. Our board takes corrective action when necessary to ensure mission compliance.

   ❏ Strongly Agree   ❏ Agree
   ❏ Disagree   ❏ Strongly Disagree

7. We periodically review, discuss, and, if necessary, amend our mission statement to ensure that it always remains current and relevant.

   ❏ Strongly Agree   ❏ Agree
   ❏ Disagree   ❏ Strongly Disagree

8. Our mission statement is more focused on the external community than it is on the institution.

   ❏ Strongly Agree   ❏ Agree
   ❏ Disagree   ❏ Strongly Disagree

9. Our board has participated in the development of and approved a strategic plan for our hospital that is consistent with and supportive of our mission statement.

   ❏ Strongly Agree   ❏ Agree
   ❏ Disagree   ❏ Strongly Disagree

10. Our board is more concerned with fulfillment of the mission than with the financial success of the organization.

    ❏ Strongly Agree   ❏ Agree
    ❏ Disagree   ❏ Strongly Disagree

Conclusion

The mission statement is the most critical document in the external relations of the organization and in the operation of the board. The mission forms the basis of the relationships with the physicians, with the community, and with other providers and organizations.

An effective board envisions the purpose of an organization and from this shapes a strategic direction to help assure that the organization achieves it. The board envisions the purpose of the organization through the mission and through the mission creates the future for the organization.

8

Strategic Planning by the Board

Strategic planning is one of the most critical responsibilities for trustees. But experience shows that it is also a task that they tend to perform the least effectively. Why? Because the board frequently focuses on and attempts to perpetuate the past rather than facilitating strategic thinking and action about the future.

That's why board members and other health care organization leaders should realize this simple truth: The health care system is undergoing rapid, sweeping changes that will affect everyone involved in it—hospitals, physicians, providers, purchasers, the government, communities, and patients. Furthermore, health care delivery is being reformed by such forces as informed and aggressive payers and employers, the rapid growth of managed care and at-risk capitation, the increasing availability of quality data, reductions in Medicare payments, and the linking of health care delivery and financing systems

Change is also being spurred by the movement away from inpatient acute care, the increasing emphasis on wellness and illness prevention, the movement toward healthy communities, and the growth and acceptance of alternative medicine.

Each of these changes is significant; together, they are revolutionary. Effective health care leaders realize that these changes are happening now, not in the distant future. Thus, health care leaders must act now.

In this environment, a failure to plan is surely a plan to fail.

What Is Strategic Planning?

Strategic planning is the process of determining what an organization should do, as well as when and how it should do it. That's why effective strategic planning involves strategic thinking, strategic decision making, and strategic action. Strategic planning has been defined as

The process of building a vision and assembling the means to carry it out.

—*Dabney G. Park Jr.*, Strategic Planning and the Nonprofit Board

An organized way of applying common sense and judgment to your hospital's decision-making process.

—*Norman H. McMillan*, Planning for Survival

Although these definitions seem to describe a simple, straightforward process, effective strategic planning involves a series of complex steps. Among other things, the process requires

- soul searching
- hard work
- thinking ahead and assessing the environment
- anticipating many alternate futures—and choosing one
- diagnosing problems
- determining solutions
- choosing a course of action—and having the courage to commit to and implement that course
- monitoring the implementation of the plan
- keeping the plan dynamic so that it responds to the changing environment and the changing needs of the organization

One of the major components of a meaningful strategic plan is an organizational vision—a sense of where the organization is heading and what it hopes to achieve. In fact, strategic planning engages the organization in a systematic process of determining what the organization is going to be and how it will get there. "Strategic planning is worthless unless there is first a strategic vision," says futurist John

Naisbitt. With the vision as the basis, the strategic planning process can then focus on how best to achieve it in light of projected environmental changes.

Questions for Discussion

A strategic planning process helps trustees to answer a set of critical questions, such as those presented below. Please consider and answer the following questions. The board members may do this individually and then discuss the answers with the entire group.

1. What is our organization's purpose or mission?
2. What is our vision for the organization's future?
3. Whom do we serve today?
4. Who are our stakeholders?
5. Whom should we serve tomorrow?
6. Which services do we provide?
7. What services should we provide?
8. What tools can we use to measure our performance?
9. How can we change our priorities if conditions change?

Exercise: Strategic Planning Development and Improvement

A common problem with many strategic planning processes arises from organizational denial: the inability or refusal of the board and other leaders to recognize the most critical issues, whether external or internal, confronting the organization. As a result, many strategic plans identify and address dozens of minor issues but fail to address the one or two absolutely crucial ones. In other words, many plans nibble at the toes of the giant rather than strike at its heart.

The entire board should discuss and agree on answers to the following questions:

1. What are the three most critical issues facing our organization?
2. What are the greatest strengths our organization can draw on to address these issues?
3. What are the greatest weaknesses our organization must overcome to address these issues?

4. What are the likely consequences of not implementing changes to address these issues for the hospital? For the physicians? For the community?

The Strategic Planning Process

Determining where to focus the finite resources of your organization is a complex task and often one that is unique to each organization. Consequently, the strategic planning process is not a set formula that each organization's board can easily follow. Each board must establish and oversee its own strategic planning process.

Nevertheless, there are steps and tasks that are common to most strategic planning processes, including the following:

1. Get organized.
   - plan to plan
   - possibly establish a planning committee
   - develop a committee charge, such as
     —work products
     —responsible parties
     —approvals
     —timetable
2. Develop or reaffirm the mission statement.
3. Develop or at least revise the vision statement.
4. Gather data and conduct an internal and external environmental assessment.
5. Analyze data and identify strategic issues.
6. Select strategic priorities and develop strategies: Make the best use of limited resources to achieve the vision.
7. Develop action plans: alternatives, recommendations, assignments of responsibilities, and time frames.
8. Determine performance measures: objective criteria, time frames.
9. Approve the strategic plan.
10. Implement the strategic plan.
11. Monitor, evaluate, and update the plan and its performance targets at least annually.

Whichever process you use to develop it, an effective strategic plan will have several essential components:

- a clear vision for the organization
- between 4 and 10 primary areas of focus, with goals and objectives for each area
- strategies to achieve the goals and objectives
- tactics to turn the strategies into action (these are often contained in action plans)

The Role of the Board

The principal responsibility for strategic planning rests with the board. Although the board does not usually conduct all of the steps involved in the planning process, it does ensure that they get accomplished appropriately. Among the board's responsibilities for strategic planning are the following:

- ensuring that a planning process is in place
- assigning responsibility to oversee the process (usually this will be assigned to a strategic planning committee of the board, but it can be assumed by the board as a whole)
- making policy decisions on the strategic direction of the organization
- ensuring that the strategic direction is consistent with the mission and vision and is appropriate to the environment
- reviewing and approving specific projects and actions to verify that they are consistent with the strategic plan
- monitoring the implementation of the strategic plan and how goals and objectives are being achieved
- modifying and updating the plan on a regular basis

It's important to remember that strategic plans are not static. Planning involves evaluating and modifying existing plans and constantly developing new ones.

Due to the accelerating pace of change in health care, time horizons of strategic plans have generally been shortened to one to three years rather than the longer time horizons of the past.

Exercise: Role Clarification

Following is a series of potential roles that a governing board might be expected to play in the strategic planning process.

Please rank (with one being the highest) each role from highest to lowest priority. Each trustee should perform this exercise individually first; then the whole board should collate and discuss the results.

Board Roles

- organize and oversee the process
- maintain the mission
- pursue the vision
- contribute community perspective
- ask questions
- set strategic direction
- set goals and priorities
- approve the strategic plan
- monitor plan implementation
- evaluate performance toward plan achievement
- maintain institutional viability
- track environmental changes
- improve community health
- oversee tactical implementation
- achieve stakeholder buy-in to the plan
- communicate the plan
- identify the strengths and weakness of the organization
- identify the opportunities and threats facing the organization
- develop goals and objectives
- examine alternative approaches and solutions

Strategic Planning Case Example

The following case example will help trustees to analyze a market situation and determine the best market position and strategic direction for Our Town General Hospital. This example can be used as part of a board retreat or, if distributed and reviewed in advance, as part of an educational component of a board meeting.

Our Town General Hospital is a 500-bed, not-for-profit community hospital serving a metropolitan area of 300,000 people. Competitors are a 350-bed community hospital, a 220-bed religiously sponsored institution with long-term care and elderly housing, and a 90-bed county-owned facility providing specialized services, including rehabilitation, chemical dependency, and women's health programs. Thirty miles away is a well-respected academic medical center with which Our Town General has a teaching affiliation.

Our Town General maintains a primarily local focus and offers a broad range of services, many of which are not well-differentiated. It is the most expensive local provider, and the community perceives the hospital as delivering high-quality service.

Although the hospital has traditionally focused on inpatient care, it was the first provider in town to diversify into outpatient services, primarily ambulatory surgery. Two years ago, the hospital also entered into a joint venture with a physician group from its medical staff to purchase and operate an MRI unit.

Our Town General's medical staff also has staff appointments at other local hospitals. Referral patterns to the hospital are moderately strong, especially for obstetrical care. Most of the medical staff falls into the 45–65 age group. Discussions are under way with key medical staff leaders about establishing a physician-hospital organization (PHO); two of Our Town General's competitors already have established PHOs.

Over the past five years, Our Town General's operating margins have been close to 4 percent. Accounts receivable now run 71 days, down from 85 days five years ago. The physical plant averages 10 years of age.

Like many communities, Our Town General's service area has a growing elderly population. The area has experienced a "baby boomlet" over the past five years, and this trend is expected to increase.

The area's employer profile is slowly changing from a manufacturing to service focus. One of the major employers in town has decided to participate in managed care.

Analysis

As a board member of Our Town General you are now participating in the hospital's strategic planning process. Management has told you that if the hospital simply maintains its current focus, its position as local market leader will likely erode and lead to continuing cost increases, reimbursement constraints, and other typical problems. How would you answer the following questions?

1. What are the three most critical issues facing Our Town General?
2. What are Our Town General's current strengths and weaknesses?
3. What key issues will the hospital face in the future? Note the potential planning implications of each issue you identify.
4. What position should Our Town General seek in the local health care delivery system?
5. Which strategic direction should the hospital adopt and why?
6. Our Town General Hospital's mission statement, approved five years ago, is as follows:

> Our Town General Hospital is a 500-bed, not-for-profit community hospital serving Our Town and adjacent communities. Our Town General provides a broad range of acute care and outpatient services and maintains a teaching focus. Our goal is to be the leading hospital in our market by delivering the highest-quality services as efficiently as possible.

> Given the strategic direction you have recommended, rewrite the mission statement to clearly and specifically indicate the hospital's purpose and identity.

Tips for Effective Governance Involvement in Strategic Planning

- Lead, don't follow. Many health care leaders are "waiting to see what's going to happen." This approach is reactive and unproductive.
- Involve key stakeholders in the planning process. These can include the board, executive management, physician leaders, community representatives, and organizations that are strategic partners with your hospital.
- Plan, then act. Do not fall prey to the "paralysis of analysis," where the constant state of gathering information and

planning precludes action by creating the false sense of security that the board is "doing something."

- Make certain that the strategic plan has the commitment of the key stakeholders before it is finalized or implemented. As Norman McMillan says, "The 25 percent plan that gets 100 percent commitment is a winner; the 100 percent plan that gets 25 percent commitment is a loser."
- Keep the strategies simple, the goals specific, and the objectives measurable.
- Place the top strategic objectives on the first or second page of every board agenda book (following the mission and vision) to enable the board to coordinate its time and attention with the strategic plan.
- Develop annual board and board committee objectives and work plans that flow from, and focus on, the strategic plan; integrate them into the board self-evaluation process.
- Use the strategic plan as a basis for the CEO performance evaluation process: develop specific CEO performance objectives based on measurable goals and objectives in the strategic plan.
- Make certain that the strategic plan focuses on the critical issues confronting your organization, not just the secondary ones.
- Most health care market conditions will require strategies for
  —cost efficiency
  —quality improvement and demonstration
  —integration of physicians
  —streamlined leadership structures
  —establishing or maintaining strategic partnerships with other organizations
  Does your plan address these issues?

A Self-Assessment Questionnaire

The following brief survey addresses the board's key roles and responsibilities in oversight of, and involvement in, the strategic planning process. It can be used as a stand-alone survey or as part of an overall board self-evaluation process. Each trustee should independently and anonymously rate the board's performance on each of the following questions.

Then compile and analyze all the responses of the trustees and discuss them with the entire board. Pay particular attention to questions with significant variation in responses (where some trustees rate board performance high and some rate it low) and those with predominately negative responses. The discussion should result in the formation of a board action plan to increase the effectiveness of its oversight and involvement in strategic planning.

1. The board takes a leadership role in organizing and overseeing the strategic planning process.

   ❑ Strongly Agree   ❑ Agree
   ❑ Disagree   ❑ Strongly Disagree

2. The board approves a strategic plan and ensures it is consistent with the organization's mission.

   ❑ Strongly Agree   ❑ Agree
   ❑ Disagree   ❑ Strongly Disagree

3. The board ensures that community perspectives and issues are addressed in the planning process.

   ❑ Strongly Agree   ❑ Agree
   ❑ Disagree   ❑ Strongly Disagree

4. Management, the medical staff, key clinical and administrative staff, community leaders and representatives, and other advisers, as appropriate, participate in our planning process.

   ❑ Strongly Agree   ❑ Agree
   ❑ Disagree   ❑ Strongly Disagree

5. The board questions planning data and assumptions and deliberates alternative strategies during our strategic planning process.

   ❑ Strongly Agree   ❑ Agree
   ❑ Disagree   ❑ Strongly Disagree

6. The board sets a strategic direction for strategic plan development.

   ❑ Strongly Agree   ❑ Agree
   ❑ Disagree   ❑ Strongly Disagree

7. The board monitors implementation of the strategic plan and evaluates accomplishment of plan goals and objectives at least annually.

❑ Strongly Agree   ❑ Agree
❑ Disagree   ❑ Strongly Disagree

8. The board periodically reviews, discusses, and, if necessary, amends the strategic plan to ensure that it remains current and relevant.

❑ Strongly Agree   ❑ Agree
❑ Disagree   ❑ Strongly Disagree

9. The board monitors the organization's programs and activities to ensure that they are consistent with the strategic plan.

❑ Strongly Agree   ❑ Agree
❑ Disagree   ❑ Strongly Disagree

10. The board takes corrective action when necessary to ensure compliance with the mission and the strategic plan.

❑ Strongly Agree   ❑ Agree
❑ Disagree   ❑ Strongly Disagree

Conclusion

The purpose of strategic planning is not only to position the organization for the future, but, in a very real sense, to create the future for the organization. For the board to effectively oversee such a process, it must break the bonds of the past to envision the future. That is why Arie P. De Geus says, "The real purpose of effective planning is not to make plans but to change the microcosm, the mental models that decision makers carry in their heads" (*Planning as Learning*). Finally, remember that "the output of planning is not a plan; the output is action!" (John Abendshien, *A Guide to the Board's Role in Strategic Business Planning*).

Information and the Effective Board

"Why did you come to Casablanca?"

"For the waters."

"But there are no waters in Casablanca!"

"I was misinformed."

—*Claude Raines quizzing Humphrey Bogart in the movie* Casablanca

Many trustees complain that while their board agenda packets are getting thicker, they feel as if they are dropping lower on the information curve. When astronomers receive data from radiotelescopes aimed at distant galaxies, they immediately categorize these data into two groups: information and noise. The noise is isolated and discarded, and the information is analyzed and acted on. So here's the fundamental question for a board: What is useful governance information, and what is noise?

Creating the Future

Health care is currently confronting what futurists call "the two curve problem." Ian Morris has explained it as follows: "A business or industry that is on a stable . . . curve confronts a second curve—'a new world order'—that transforms the existing business or industry and threatens to replace or surpass the original curve. . . . The two-curve problem presents difficult choices for [boards] because the pace of change is

92

uncertain and the degree to which the second curve will sur-pass the first is unclear. Compounding the dilemma, the first curve is usually very profitable and the second curve very risky."[1]

When the first curve yields to the second, everything changes, especially the board's information needs. The incentives under managed care, for example, are diametrically opposed to those of fee for service. A board that bases its deliberations and decisions on a fee-for-service information structure while attempting to lead its organization in a managed care environment will invariably lead its organization to failure.

When times were relatively stable and prosperous, a typical board spent most of its time monitoring the past. The information the board received, and its agenda, were largely devoted to reviews of what happened last month, last quarter, or last year. This type of "looking in the rearview mirror" governance information tends to perpetuate the past rather than prepare a board to address the future.

Effective boards control the information they receive and how they spend their time. When approaching a new curve or paradigm, or in its early stages, a board should spend most of its time deliberating and planning the future. Talking about the past (monitoring) should be reduced to no more than 25 percent of a board's time, and talking about and creating the future (planning, setting policy, and making decisions) should consume most, or about 75 percent, of a board's time. Boards must drive their organizations by spending most of their time looking out the windshield, not in the rearview mirror.

Questions for Discussion

Please consider and answer the following questions and exercises. This may be done by each trustee and then discussed with the whole board.

---

1. Ian Morrison, Ph.D., "The Two-Curve Problem: High-Risk Challenges Face Those Who Plan a Hospital's Future," *Health Management Quarterly* 16, no. 1 (first qtr. 1994): 11.

1. Mentally divide the information presented to your board in agenda materials and during board meetings into two categories: information about the past and information about the future. What percentage of your board's information relates to the past? What percentage relates to the future? Is this division appropriate? If not, how should it be changed?

2. Many types of information that were crucial under the old curve are irrelevant under the new curve. For example, accounts receivable is important financial information under a fee-for-service system but is largely, if not entirely, irrelevant under a capitated payment system. What other types of governance information were crucial under the old curve but will be of minimal or no importance under the new curve? What new types of governance information will likely be required under the new curve?

Information Problems

A health care organization uses three types of information: management, clinical, and governance. If a board is given management information, it will manage. If a board is given clinical information, it will attempt to practice medicine. Boards respond to the information they are given.

That's why it is critical that boards be given governance information. Unfortunately, many boards do not receive this information in their agenda materials. Instead, they get operational detail, warmed-over management reports, and detailed clinical information.

Here are some common flaws and weaknesses in providing information and reports to boards:

- Reports and information do not flow from or support the explicitly defined role of the board on the issue.
- There are no guidelines regarding what information should be reported to the board or how it should be reported.
- Reports provide data, such as clinical indicators, but not information, such as trends or projections.

- Meeting minutes are used as a vehicle for providing information to the board (that is, the board finance committee minutes are used as the financial report to the board).
- Too much material is presented in the reports.
- Governance reports are simply retitled management or medical staff information.
- Ineffective report formats blunt the board's understanding of important information.
- Thick board agenda packets are distributed to board members so close to the scheduled meeting that they have no time to read all the material.
- Significant amounts of informational materials are routinely distributed to board members for review at the board meeting.

Information Control

Much information provided to a board reflects issues that have been considered by another, subordinate group in the organization (such as a board or management committee). In this situation board members should usually receive a summary distillation of the information that the group has already considered.

For a graphic example of this point, consider figures 9-1 through 9-3. Imagine that a system chief financial officer (CFO) is addressing a particular issue, say, days cash on hand. The CFO might consider 25 pages of information on this issue. Now the CEO probably also considers this issue. If both the CEO and the CFO consider the same issue, what then is the difference in their jobs? The difference is authority and oversight and level of detail reviewed. So the CEO might see only 10 pages of information on days cash on hand.

Next, a report on this topic is prepared for the board finance committee (BFC). If the BFC sees 25 pages of information on the subject, the committee will, in effect, be doing the CFO's job. So the BFC might see only one page of information on days cash on hand. This same issue might also be reported to the board, but the board might be provided

FIGURE 9-1. Effective Governance Information Flow

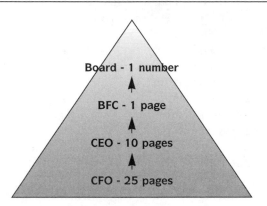

FIGURE 9-2. Ineffective Governance Information Flow

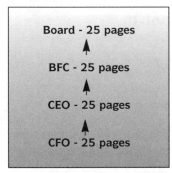

FIGURE 9-3. Dysfunctional Governance Information Flow

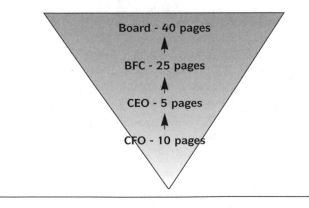

with only one number, along with target points or upper and lower control limits of performance.

Of course, if the one number or indicator received by the board is outside the target range, the board could then ask for more information. This "drilling down" for information is done by a board only when the governance indicators warrant it.

Unfortunately, many boards do not follow this process. Ineffective boards follow the process graphically depicted in figure 9-2. This, however, is not the worst example of information flow. That dubious honor goes to figure 9-3. In figure 9-3, the board is actually seeing more data than the groups below it need to do their jobs. This is not only ineffective, it is dysfunctional.

Effective governance is facilitated not only by the amount of information the board receives but also by its format. For most boards, a picture is worth a thousand words. Graphic displays of data, showing patterns or trends of performance over time, help condense and summarize a variety of data into one simple display. Graphic reports that not only show performance over time but also provide upper and lower performance thresholds turn raw data into useful information and become tools that help boards interpret and question performance variations.

Organizations that want their information technology to help provide useful organization-wide governance information need to invest in technology that can respond to a specific request for information and then organize the data to show performance over time. Data-mining capability also can assist a board to drill down into an organization's complex database to gather further information to expediently answer questions about performance variation.

As boards review proposals for investment in information systems, they should determine whether the proposed technology can generate the type of organization-wide data and reports that will not only assist with operating, but with governing the entire health care system as well.

Questions for Discussion

1. Of the three models of governance information flow, which is most typical of the way that information flows to your board?

2. Does the way information flows to your board vary by topic or by committee? If so, which topics or content areas have the best information flow (such as figure 9-1). Which are like figure 9-2? Which, if any, are like figure 9-3? Why?

3. Are the same reports, with the same level of detail, usually provided to more than one governance structure?

4. Does your board receive information primarily in graphic or written format? What information, if any, is presented graphically? How do the board's questions, deliberations, or actions differ depending on the format of the information that it receives?

5. Has your board recently reviewed or approved a request for investment in organization-wide information capability? Will the information capability your organization plans to acquire support the level of performance monitoring and evaluation required for effective decision making and planning in an increasingly complex environment?

Types of Information

In times of change, the job of leadership is to make others within the organization uncomfortable, to move them along the process of change. To do this, boards must first make themselves uncomfortable. A key technique for a board to push itself outside its comfort zone is to demand new types and formats of information. This technique helps a board to stretch itself into the understanding and mastery of important new areas, as well as to send clear messages throughout the organization that change is here.

Effective governance information will increasingly involve an external focus, such as market and governmental trends, as opposed to an exclusively internal focus.

Exercise: Governance Information

Please review the following categories of potential governance information and answer the questions that follow.

- financial performance
- competitive position and market power
- CEO performance evaluation
- inpatient clinical quality and cost efficiency
- outpatient clinical quality and cost efficiency
- enrolled population (covered lives) quality and access to health care indicators
- medical staff credentialing
- representation of stakeholder interests
- physician relations
- physician integration
- affiliation, alliances, mergers, joint ventures
- community health assessment and improvement
- federal legislative trends for Medicare reimbursement
- regulatory compliance reports
- governance performance evaluation
- building and grounds reports
- human resources reports
- strategic planning

1. Which of the preceding categories of governance information does your board most often receive and review? Which does your board receive least often? Which categories, if any, does your board never receive? Why?
2. What categories of governance information are you most comfortable with? What types of information are you least comfortable with? Why? What about your board as a whole?
3. If your board could receive only five categories of information, which would you choose? Why?

Tips on Providing Effective Information to the Board

- Informational reports to the board should be brief and in graphic format whenever possible.
- Any narrative reports provided to a board should be prefaced by an executive summary.
- All information provided to a board should directly relate to the organization's strategy and goals, as well as support the achievement of the board's annual goals and objectives.

- Meeting minutes should never be used as the primary vehicle for providing information to a board.
- The board should annually develop and select a series of topic-specific indicators (for example, quality, finance, and executive performance) that will be routinely presented to the board.
- The board should set thresholds or target levels for each indicator. If the indicator is within established limits, the board will not need to review it. If an indicator trend line has approached or exceeded an upper or lower limit, the board should devote attention to it.
- Indicators, along with upper and lower limits or thresholds, should be presented to the board in graphic format. That facilitates a quick review and provides the board with a big-picture view of the issues.
- An annual calendar should be developed for reporting routine or required information to the board (such as medical staff credentialing, quality reporting, CEO performance evaluation, and board reports required by external regulators).
- The quality, quantity, format, and effectiveness of governance information should be included as part of the annual board self-evaluation.
- The board should ensure that its organization has the information system support necessary to assist with required levels of planning and decision making.
- Governance information should be tailored to lead the business and future focus of the organization, not to follow behind it.

A Self-Assessment Questionnaire

The following brief survey addresses the appropriate types and level of detail of information sent to the board. It can be used as a stand-alone survey or as part of an overall board self-evaluation process.

Each trustee should independently and anonymously rate the board's performance on each of the following questions. Compile and analyze all the responses of the members and discuss them with the entire board. Pay particular attention to questions with significant variation in responses and those with predominately negative responses.

1. The information the board receives is complete and adequate for board-level discussion and decision making.

   ❑ Strongly Agree   ❑ Agree
   ❑ Somewhat Disagree   ❑ Disagree

2. Review of governance information that monitors the organization's past events and activities is confined to no more than 25 percent of the board's meeting time.

   ❑ Strongly Agree   ❑ Agree
   ❑ Somewhat Disagree   ❑ Disagree

3. The information that is provided to board members is not limited only to acute, inpatient care but also includes information and indicators relating to outpatient care, community health, managed care, and other areas reflecting the probable future activities, focus, and business mix of the organization.

   ❑ Strongly Agree   ❑ Agree
   ❑ Somewhat Disagree   ❑ Disagree

4. Performance indicators (quality, finance, and so on) are mostly presented to the board in graphic format, with goals, thresholds, or upper and lower control limits included on the graph.

   ❑ Strongly Agree   ❑ Agree
   ❑ Somewhat Disagree   ❑ Disagree

5. The information the board receives is tailored to the organization's strategic plan, as well as the board's annual goals, objectives, and priorities.

   ❑ Strongly Agree   ❑ Agree
   ❑ Somewhat Disagree   ❑ Disagree

6. Board agenda materials are sent out far enough in advance for board members to review them thoroughly.

   ❑ Strongly Agree   ❑ Agree
   ❑ Somewhat Disagree   ❑ Disagree

7. I review all agenda materials thoroughly before each
   board meeting.

   ❏ Strongly Agree   ❏ Agree
   ❏ Somewhat Disagree   ❏ Disagree

8. Board members are given regular information and access
   to education programs, key health care issues, and board
   roles and responsibilities.

   ❏ Strongly Agree   ❏ Agree
   ❏ Somewhat Disagree   ❏ Disagree

9. The board annually reviews and revises the content,
   amount, and format of the information it receives.

   ❏ Strongly Agree   ❏ Agree
   ❏ Somewhat Disagree   ❏ Disagree

Conclusion

Effective boards must become change masters. To accomplish
this, they must explore new ideas and approaches and pursue
new strategies for their organizations. But first a board must
explicitly control and structure the information it receives to
ensure that it is relevant to the organization's future. Boards
that do this effectively will be best prepared to lead their
organizations into the future; those that do not will be con-
demned to govern within the paradigms of the past.

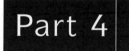

Part 4

*Board
Relations*

CEO Evaluation and Compensation

At a recent meeting, the board of one hospital in a two-hospital town said it would be a good idea if its facility took the lead in assessing and improving the community's health. Interpreting this as a board directive, the CEO began allocating his time and other organizational resources to the task.

But several months later, the trustees complained that the CEO wasn't "sticking to his knitting"; they saw organizational priorities shifting away from the inpatient, hospital focus. Further, many trustees were uncomfortable with their CEO's participation in a community health improvement partnership with the other hospital. So the board challenged the CEO on these activities.

Stunned by the criticism, the CEO shot back, "I'm simply doing what you told me to do; you gave me a specific directive." Surprised, the chairman said: "We never told you to do that; we were only thinking out loud." The board told the CEO to stop focusing resources on a health assessment and to refocus on "doing what needs to be done."

"Precisely what is that?" the CEO asked. Replied the chairman, "If you don't know, maybe we need a CEO who does."

This story illustrates the key relationship between board and CEO and how it is often framed by implicit assumptions and unspoken expectations about relative roles and performance objectives. That's why the board-CEO relationship frequently is not as stable or effective as it could or needs to be.

It's clearly not the trustees' role to manage or operate the organization on a daily basis, but it is their function to monitor how it is managed. This means that in addition to working with the CEO as a leadership partner, the board must monitor and evaluate the CEO's performance as an employee.

Purposes and Benefits of the CEO Evaluation Process

The CEO performance evaluation is a crucial board function. Yet, as important as the process is, many boards are uncomfortable with this responsibility. An effective CEO evaluation is planned, deliberate, objective, and fair. Although the evaluation is a governance function, it involves interaction between the board and CEO in all phases of the process.

There's more to CEO evaluation than simply extending or terminating the CEO's employment. Other, equally important purposes and benefits of the evaluation process include

- linking compensation to CEO performance and providing an objective basis for recognizing and rewarding excellent performance
- focusing the CEO's activities on the organization's mission and strategic plan
- providing a mechanism to assess how effectively the CEO has implemented the policies and decisions of the board
- identifying problems with board policies and decisions early on, thus allowing for timely changes
- providing a basis for future CEO performance expectations as well as board performance objectives and goals
- facilitating coordination and teamwork among the organization's leadership
- creating a formal system to develop the CEO both professionally and personally
- clarifying the practical distinction between governance and management
- reaffirming, revising, or clarifying the board's expectations of the CEO
- fostering a formal "expectations exchange," where, through mutual discussion and negotiation, the board clarifies its

expectations of the CEO and the CEO clarifies his or her
expectations of the board

- protecting the CEO against the considerable risk associated with doing his or her job properly
- establishing parameters for CEO performance that enable
  the board to retain and reward the CEO with a raise, quickly and appropriately terminate the CEO's employment, or
  provide constructive feedback regarding CEO performance
  that is not quite up to par

Keeping this list in mind will help both boards and CEOs
establish or redesign the executive evaluation process around
four main goals:

1. appropriate assessment and reward of CEO performance
2. linkage of executive performance to the organization's
   goals
3. CEO growth and development
4. strengthening board/CEO relations

Start-Up Tools

To design an effective CEO evaluation process, an organization board needs

- a clearly defined vision, mission, and set of values
- an up-to-date strategic plan with clearly specified organizational goals and objectives, along with stated measures
  of what it would mean to achieve those goals
- a current, written job description for the CEO that includes
  the organization's goals and objectives as outlined in the
  strategic plan
- a current, written job description for the board of trustees
- a shared understanding of the purposes of the CEO evaluation

The formal evaluation process must be deliberate and
fair. Although the process should be as objective as possible,
it will always involve some degree of subjectivity. Just be
sure that you recognize the subjective elements and weight
them appropriately in relation to the objective elements.

Although CEO evaluations are frequently conducted on an annual basis, the actual process should be ongoing, allowing for continuous feedback to the CEO on his or her performance and modification of performance objectives. Finally, the evaluation process should cover every aspect of the CEO's employment.

Elements of the Evaluation Process

Although each evaluation process may reflect unique aspects of leadership character and style as well as the organization's values and goals, effective processes often share key elements.

Executive Compensation Philosophy

Both the evaluation and its implementation should flow from a written compensation philosophy that is based on the organization's short- and long-term strategic objectives. The philosophy should address such issues as expectations of the CEO, organization, and other key stakeholders; mix and balance of fixed (salary and benefits) and variable (incentives) compensation; the relationship of performance to the total compensation package; the relationship of risk to incentives; and the use of performance standards linked to expectations and comparisons with strategic competitors in the industry.

Who Takes Responsibility?

More and more health care boards are vesting responsibility for CEO evaluation and compensation with a formal compensation committee of the board. Making such a committee responsible for evaluating the CEO and other key executives provides a depth and continuity of focus that helps ensure that the process is comprehensive, up-to-date, and functioning properly for all participants.

Monitoring, Review, and Revision

The compensation committee should report to the full board at least annually on its ongoing review of the CEO and revision of objectives to ensure that all trustees understand and support the process.

Evaluation and Compensation: A Case Study

The board of Peak Hospital and Medical Center had just completed a strategic planning retreat. The board had expanded the hospital's mission to focus on responsibility for community health and the need for developing partnerships with other providers and community organizations. The chairman of the Peak board was pleased with the outcome of the retreat and wanted to ensure that the hospital turned this mission into action. He shared his concerns over lunch with a colleague who was on the board of a *Fortune* 1,000 company in town. The colleague related a story of his own.

> A few years ago our company was faced with several issues that were becoming critical to our survival. Our board realized that unless these issues were addressed and monitored vigilantly, our company would lose its competitive position. It was clear that we needed to establish some specific goals for these key issues and invest responsibility for achieving them in our company's CEO and management team.
>
> Our board worked through its compensation committee to establish goals and timetables and to set up a periodic review process to ensure that goals and performance remained on target. The committee also looked at other companies in our industry to determine specific types of compensation and incentive packages that could help motivate and sustain the type of performance we wanted.
>
> We set up an annual incentive program tied to progress toward our three-year goals and a payout at the end based on goal achievement. We made the committee responsible not only for monitoring progress and evaluating the CEO, but also for providing coaching and development opportunities.
>
> We ended up exceeding our three-year targets and increasing our market share. And we now have a group of committed, enthusiastic executives who gear

their performance toward meeting the organization's long-term goals and sharing in the organization's success.

After lunch, the hospital board chairman reflected on his own board's CEO evaluation process. It consisted of an annual review of the CEO's performance by the chairman and vice chairman, based on a summary of activities and accomplishments prepared by the CEO. The CEO usually received a salary increase and a bonus if the hospital's bottom line was reasonably healthy. But the chairman realized that fulfilling the revised mission would require different expectations of the CEO and management team and new levels of performance as well.

Questions for Discussion

1. What aspects of the *Fortune* 1,000 company's executive evaluation and compensation process could be useful to the hospital?
2. Who should be involved in reevaluating the hospital's executive evaluation and compensation process?
3. Who should be responsible for CEO evaluation and compensation review?
4. What goals should the board establish with the hospital's executive team to ensure that the organization focuses on achieving the mission?
5. How can the board make sure that the evaluation and compensation process continues to function effectively?
6. How might the hospital extend the evaluation and compensation process to ensure that the entire organization is focused on achieving strategic goals?

Mastering Change

A series of paradigm shifts of unprecedented proportions is occurring in health care (see figure 10-1). When a paradigm shifts, everything changes; the old rules for success no longer work. In fact, following old rules usually causes failure in the new reality.

Hospital leaders traditionally resist change. That's why they are usually swept along or over by change and rarely influence, control, manage, or direct the change that will dictate their future.

Effective CEOs must become change masters. To do this, they must be open to a series of structured inquiries, a raising of key questions that will spur them to explore new ideals and approaches and put forth new objectives for their organizations. Perhaps the best mechanism with which to accomplish this is the CEO performance evaluation and objectives-setting process.

FIGURE 10-1. Paradigms and CEO Evaluation

Following are several of the paradigm shifts that are occurring in health care. Please review them and use them to address the questions that follow.

From	To
A focus on facilities	A focus on services
Hospitals	Integrated delivery systems
A focus on acute care illness	Continuum of care, prevention
Delivery of care	Delivery and financing of care
Focus on the patient	Focus on community health and wellness
Market share as admissions	Market share as covered lives, physicians
Managing stability (reactive)	Leading change (proactive)
Cumbersome, slow decision making	Streamlined, rapid decision making

1. Which of these changing directions in health care has your board and CEO specifically addressed via new or modified CEO performance objectives?

2. How has the relative weight given to each of your CEO's performance objectives changed to reflect any of the above transitions?

3. If your CEO performance objectives have not been modified in the past several years, what is the explicit rationale for maintaining the "old" CEO performance objectives and evaluation process?

CEO Employment Contracts

Chief executives often need to take action that is risky to both their careers and the organization. Initiating aggressive action can generate turmoil and uncertainty in the organization and community, as well as bitter resistance among key stakeholders, such as physician groups.

If the CEO is unsure of the board's support or doesn't know what the board expects, then he or she is more likely to play it safe, to favor short-term stability over long-term organizational survival. To help protect CEOs against the considerable risk of doing their jobs properly, boards should provide them with written employment contracts.

Contracts not only allow CEOs to take risks but also reward and help retain successful executives. A one-to-two-year severance package, supplemental or accelerated retirement, and other benefits can help provide the risk/reward combination that supports the CEO and the organization's objectives.

Community Health and CEO Performance Expectations

Responsibility for the health of a community and the need to manage the delivery of health care against fixed payment require new CEO performance objectives and evaluation criteria. A comprehensive set of evaluation criteria should reflect the CEO's responsibilities for both internal and external results and relationships.

Topics/criteria for CEO evaluation should include

- organizational results
  —financial measures
  —market share
  —quality
  —achievement of strategic objectives
  —daily operations
- community health
  —community health status
  —amount of charitable care
  —health promotion, screening, education

- organizational relationships and culture
  —individual and professional skills
  —medical staff relations
  —relationships with other physician groups
  —board relations
  —employee relations
  —clear organizational direction
  —clarity and efficiency of strategic planning
  —community relations
  —management development
  —legislative advocacy
  —payer-purchaser relationships
  —affiliations/partnerships
- individual and professional skills
  —management style: autocratic versus participative
  —interpersonal skills and influence: consensus building
  —managerial effectiveness: delegation, group leadership, empowerment
  —problem solving: creativity, use of expertise, depth, vision
  —personal effectiveness: self-confidence and control, energy, flexibility, ethical behavior

---

Exercise: Establishing or Updating CEO Evaluation Criteria

This exercise may be conducted by the board committee responsible for CEO evaluation, with results shared and discussed with the full board.

1. Which criteria do the board currently use to evaluate the CEO?
2. Do current criteria reflect or expand on the categories listed above?
3. Are your criteria weighted to reflect the board's CEO performance priorities?
4. How would you weight the criteria mentioned above?
5. How often are your criteria reviewed or revised?
6. Does the CEO participate in establishing or updating evaluation criteria? If not, which process could be put in place to involve the CEO?

The Board's Role in CEO Evaluation: A Self-Assessment Questionnaire

The questions in the following brief survey address the board's key roles and responsibilities for overseeing the CEO evaluation process. This survey can be used as a stand-alone survey or as part of an overall board self-evaluation process.

Each trustee should independently and anonymously rate the board's performance on each of the following questions. Compile and analyze all the responses and discuss them with the entire board. Pay particular attention to questions with significant variation in responses (where some trustees rate board performance high and some rate it low), and those with predominately negative responses. Note: The CEO should also complete the questionnaire and participate in the discussion. The discussion should result in an action plan to improve CEO performance.

1. Has our board approved a written job description for the position of CEO?

   ❏ Yes   ❏ No   ❏ Don't Know

2. Does the board have an employment contract with the CEO?

   ❏ Yes   ❏ No   ❏ Don't Know

3. The board has a formal CEO evaluation process that includes written annual performance objectives.

   ❏ Strongly Agree   ❏ Agree
   ❏ Disagree   ❏ Strongly Disagree

4. The board reviews and modifies the CEO performance objectives to ensure that they are consistent with the mission, strategy, and organizational objectives of the organization.

   ❏ Strongly Agree   ❏ Agree
   ❏ Disagree   ❏ Strongly Disagree

5. We periodically review, discuss, and, if necessary, modify the CEO performance objectives to ensure that they are current and reflect changing market conditions and board expectations.

   ❏ Strongly Agree   ❏ Agree
   ❏ Disagree   ❏ Strongly Disagree

6. We provide ongoing feedback to the CEO on his/her performance relative to the performance objectives.

   ❏ Strongly Agree   ❏ Agree
   ❏ Disagree   ❏ Strongly Disagree

7. Renewal of the CEO's employment contract is contingent on a performance review and based on preestablished criteria.

   ❏ Strongly Agree   ❏ Agree
   ❏ Disagree   ❏ Strongly Disagree

8. The CEO performance objectives reflect a strong commitment to the community and to the assessment and improvement of the community's health.

   ❏ Strongly Agree   ❏ Agree
   ❏ Disagree   ❏ Strongly Disagree

9. At least 20 percent of the weighted CEO performance objectives focus on assessing and improving community health.

   ❏ Strongly Agree   ❏ Agree
   ❏ Disagree   ❏ Strongly Disagree

10. Our current CEO performance objectives and evaluation process are focused to help us lead our organization effectively into the 21st century and to achieve our strategic plan.

    ❏ Strongly Agree   ❏ Agree
    ❏ Disagree   ❏ Strongly Disagree

11. The board takes a leadership rule in organizing and overseeing the CEO evaluation process.

❏ Strongly Agree   ❏ Agree
❏ Disagree   ❏ Strongly Disagree

Conclusion

A meaningful CEO evaluation process is a key component of shared leadership. Effective boards and CEOs recognize this by participating in a formal process of CEO evaluation (as well as the related process of board self-evaluation). A comprehensive evaluation process not only builds stronger leadership relationships but, when tied to strategic goals, can be a powerful motivator of organizational success.

11

New Relationships with Physicians: An Overview for Trustees

The typical medical staff organization is insufficient to cope with radically changed circumstances. New forms are necessary to help physicians and hospitals become indispensable in a market that no longer wants to purchase health care in a piecemeal manner from a bunch of different entities moving in different directions in different ways.

—*Robert Derzon,* The Corporatization of Healthcare Delivery, *1989*

As resources become increasingly scarce and tightly controlled, health care organizations must integrate their services with those of other providers in order to use those resources more efficiently and to reduce costs relentlessly.

One of the most critical and difficult aspects of this integration involves physicians. To effect the level of integration that is needed, new relationships and partnerships between providers and physicians must be created—even as the old models are destroyed.

Why is integration with doctors so critical to the success of the health care organization as well as the physicians? The answer comes from a core principle of business economics that states that the fundamental means of production must be controlled by the business. This is absolutely essential if the business has any chance of controlling costs and thriving in a more efficient market.

What, precisely, does controlling the fundamental means of production mean? Consider another industry, aerospace. The fundamental means of production of an aerospace company are its engineers, who design and build its products. The company depends on its engineers' creativity to design products and on their efficiency to produce them. If the engineers are inefficient and unproductive, the company suffers; as the market tightens, the company goes out of business.

An aerospace company "controls" its fundamental means of production, its engineers, by employing them. As employees, the engineers are under the direct control of the company, which can then control their performance with incentive and compensation plans, among other means.

Doctors are the fundamental means of production of a health care organization. They create the "product." In fact, they spend their organization's resources when they order tests, procedures, and treatments. If the costs of those tests and treatments exceed the reimbursement received for them, the organization suffers financially.

As the market tightens, the organization will decline and fail. Consequently, in an efficient market, the work produced by physicians must be controlled by the health care organization. Which means that the physicians must be controlled.

Health care, however, is coming out of a 30-year period that rewarded inefficiency handsomely; the more inefficient a health care organization was, the more money it made. Therefore, health care organizations had no incentive to seek control over their physicians, because to do so would increase efficiency and decrease revenue. As a result, hospitals and other health care organizations today find themselves in bizarre relationships with their fundamental means of production: Not only do they not control them, they are, to varying degrees, controlled by them.

Health care organizations are dependent upon physicians for the vast majority of their revenues. Employment of doctors has increased, particularly among recent medical school graduates and those who want to trade the headache of increasing expenses and declining revenues in private practice for more stable employment income. Still, most physicians do not work for a hospital or system. The vast majority are independent contractors associated with the organization through weak and transitory linkages, such as membership on the medical staff.

How health care organizations achieve this control (doctors as owners, partners, employees, stakeholders) is still a matter of great debate. Many models are being tested in the market, ranging from loose collaborative partnerships to full integration with doctors through practice acquisition and employment. Several of these models are described here.

Integration Models

One approach to hospital-physician partnerships is the cooperative. This loose, voluntary form of collaboration between a hospital or health system and a number of doctors enables the parties involved to enter into joint ventures. While it is not viewed as a strong way to affect clinical outcomes and create alignment among all parties, this model can build mutual respect and reliance.

A second model, the management services organization (MSO), can be formed between a health care organization and a multispecialty physician group or several physician practices. Each practice remains independent but is linked through common management, which provides a core of services that physicians purchase. These services can include

- billing
- information system acquisition and installation
- staffing
- staff training and development
- managed care contract negotiation and compliance
- other office management functions

Advantages of this model are

- facilitation and coordination of referrals and consistent practice patterns
- potential for economies of scale in management

- integration of information systems to facilitate the flow of patient information between physician offices and hospital settings
- a coordinated approach to the market
- few changes in practice relationships

Disadvantages can include

- the potential for competition among physicians in the organization
- suboptimal distribution of practice types and locations
- limited influence over improvement of practice patterns
- limited risk management

Physician-hospital organizations (PHOs) bring hospitals or health systems together with selected groups of physicians to enable joint contracting under managed care and collaboration to demonstrate and enhance quality of care. While PHOs are growing in number across the country, success to date has been limited. Modest gains have been reported in managed care contracting, improving relationships with community doctors, sharing financial risk, collaborating with the medical staff, and improving quality of care. But few PHOs have attempted or achieved cost management or reduction.

Ultimately, success for PHOs under managed care will depend on their ability to assume the financial risk inherent in capitated contracts and to address such issues as

- grouping doctors into subpanels
- assigning risk among primary care physicians, specialists, and the hospital
- developing economic credentialing criteria that link physician practice patterns with cost-effective resource use

The medical foundation model involves a hospital establishing a not-for-profit corporate foundation, which in turn purchases the nonphysician assets of a group of physicians and provides the support necessary to administer the practice. Under this model, doctors form a professional services corporation that contracts with the foundation to provide all physician services.

Advantages of this model include

- the ability to control outcomes and costs and therefore manage risk
- liquidity for physicians
- operating economies
- access to patient information and patients through managed care

The downsides include loss of control for physicians over the business aspects of their practices and the need to cooperate as a group.

A fully integrated health system model is often achieved by purchasing physician practices (and subsequent employment of those physicians) or by establishing a staff-model HMO. This model promises the greatest opportunity for hospitals and physicians to respond together to the market, to manage outcomes, and to rationalize resource allocation. While doctors still tend to favor a degree of autonomy over total integration with hospitals, continuing market pressure for effective cost control and the ability to demonstrate quality and performance are moving hospitals and physicians closer together.

Regardless of the relationship model selected, to be truly integrated, an integrated delivery system (IDS) must share risk and align incentives with its doctors. Further, integration with physicians must achieve and maintain a proper balance between primary care physicians and specialists.

Questions for Discussion

1. What type(s) of relationship(s) does your hospital or health system have with physicians? Which relationship or structure involves the largest number of physicians? Which relationship is the most important to your organization?
2. What percentage of the doctors associated with your health care organization are employed by it? What percentage are independent contractors? What have been the advantages and disadvantages of each type of relationship from both the organization's and physicians' perspectives?

3. Consider the environment and market in which your organization now operates. What goals, needs, or incentives are common to both your organization and its physicians? Where do your needs and incentives differ from those of the doctors? How might your organization and its physicians come together to achieve mutual goals?
4. What level of integration between your hospital and its doctors do you think will be necessary to be successful in your market? What level of integration do you think will be achievable? How?

Possible Problems with Alliances

Alliances that combine hospital and physician services have the greatest potential to deliver a seamless continuum of cost-effective care. But experts acknowledge that a variety of factors will affect whether and how organizations and physicians collaborate successfully. Such factors include market conditions, characteristics of the organization, a hospital's existing relationships with its physicians, and physician attitudes.

The following exercise can help your board assess the organization's current relationship with physicians and identify potential problems that could affect the readiness for an alliance.

Exercise: Identifying Early Warning Signs of Trouble in Your Relationship with Physicians

---

Review the following warning signs and then answer the questions at the end of the section.

- Communication breakdowns inhibit the flow and accuracy of information between the various physician groups and the board.
- There is insufficient physician membership on the board of the health care organization or system.
- Physician representatives on the IDS board are drawn from hospital medical staff leadership instead of from the leadership of one or several of the newer physician entities, such as a PHO, MSO, or physician organization.

- The roles and responsibilities of the system board, physician boards, or other leadership groups are not well defined or clearly understood.
- No joint leadership retreats are held.
- No meaningful training program for new physician-group leaders exists.
- There are significant differences in the level of organizational maturity between the health care organization or system board and the physician organization board.
- Dysfunctional personalities tend to be elected to leadership positions in the physician groups or on the organizational board.
- There are no common goals shared by the hospital or system board and the physician organization board(s).
- There is only one model available for physicians to relate to or integrate with the organization.

Questions for Discussion

1. Which, if any, of the previous warning signs does your organization or board manifest?
2. What other warning signs of impending trouble in the relationship with physicians can you identify?
3. Of the preceding list, as well as the answers to question 2 above, which warning signs do you consider the most dangerous and the least dangerous? Why?
4. What mechanisms does your health care organization have in place to monitor its relationships with doctors on an ongoing basis?
5. What mechanisms or processes does your organization have in place to address potential problems?

Tips for Building Positive Relationships with Physicians

Health care organizations can take a variety of steps to assess and strengthen their relationships with doctors.

- Conduct a structured assessment of the current relationship between the health care organization and the physicians. Use the assessment to identify strengths to build upon and weaknesses that need improvement.

- Provide assistance to help physician groups develop organizational maturity. There can be no common cause between an organization and physician groups until both parties understand and accept each other's roles and responsibilities and work toward a common vision.
- Improve communication between the health care organization board and the board of the physician group(s). Methods include having doctors on the health care organization's board, joint planning activities and leadership retreats, and planned social events.
- Address conflict in the earliest possible stage.
- Monitor the relationship and look for opportunities to constantly improve it.

The Board-Physician Relationship: A Self-Assessment Questionnaire

The following brief survey addresses the board's roles and responsibilities in overseeing the development and success of new models of physician integration and partnerships. It can be used as a stand-alone survey or as part of an overall board self-evaluation process.

Have each trustee independently and anonymously rate the board's performance on each of the following questions. Compile and analyze all responses and discuss them with the entire board. Pay particular attention to questions with significant variation in responses (where some trustees rate board performance high and some rate it low) and those with predominately negative responses.

1. Does the organization have a formal physician integration strategy that has been approved by the board?

   ❏ Yes   ❏ No

2. Does your organization have a mechanism to negotiate combined payments to your hospital and doctors? (For example, could your organization accept a single payment that covered all physician services and those provided by the organization?)

   ❏ Yes   ❏ No

3. Other than representatives of the hospital medical staff, are any doctors on your board voting members?

❏ Yes   ❏ No

4. Do you have several different mechanisms and models for doctors to link with the organization, including one that involves sharing economic risk?

❏ Yes   ❏ No

5. Your board takes a leadership role in overseeing the various integration relationships with physicians.

❏ Strongly Agree   ❏ Agree
❏ Disagree   ❏ Strongly Disagree

6. There is a common understanding of the relative roles and responsibilities of the system board, hospital board, and physician organization boards among all the organization's leaders.

❏ Strongly Agree   ❏ Agree
❏ Disagree   ❏ Strongly Disagree

7. Your organization conducts joint educational and social activities for board members, executives, and physician leaders.

❏ Strongly Agree   ❏ Agree
❏ Disagree   ❏ Strongly Disagree

8. Your organization provides physician leaders with an orientation to their leadership roles and responsibilities, as well as ongoing leadership development opportunities.

❏ Strongly Agree   ❏ Agree
❏ Disagree   ❏ Strongly Disagree

9. Doctors are part of the organization's management structure and act as liaisons with the medical staff and other physician entities.

❏ Strongly Agree   ❏ Agree
❏ Disagree   ❏ Strongly Disagree

10. A variety of communication mechanisms exist between the organization and physicians; they are used to promote ongoing dialogue and information exchange as well as to help monitor relationships and identify issues that need attention.

   ❏ Strongly Agree   ❏ Agree
   ❏ Disagree   ❏ Strongly Disagree

Conclusion

The dynamics of today's health care marketplace pose significant challenges and pressures that demand closer, more effective working relationships between health care organizations and their physicians. Unfortunately, these pressures and challenges often polarize the two groups rather than unite them. This paradoxical effect has the potential to do great damage to health care organizations. Developing and maintaining a productive relationship between the organization and its doctors is crucial to achieving the organization's mission, providing patient care that is consistent in cost and quality, and ensuring the health care organization's continued viability.

The Board-Physician Partnership: Enhancing Leadership Potential

Leaders are made, not born.

Stop and reflect on some of history's great leaders and you'll see the truth in the above statement. Julius Caesar didn't burst onto the scene as one of Rome's greatest emperors but spent years in the provinces in lesser administrative and military positions, learning and perfecting the skills and knowledge he would someday need to take control of the republic. William Wallace, the Scotsman better known as Braveheart, might never have led his countrymen in revolt if he hadn't been raised abroad and gained an education and awareness that there was more to life than poverty and oppression. Even Moses wandered 40 years in the desert before leading his people to the Promised Land.

Whether it's education, training, life experience, or a combination of all three, successful leaders grow into their roles. They achieve competency, and sometimes greatness, if they continue to learn along the way. Conversely, those who are thrust into positions of leadership without preparation or an opportunity to acquire some tools for the task are often doomed to failure or hardship. President Ulysses S. Grant comes to mind, as do the troubled presidencies of Lech Walesa of Poland and Vaclav Havel of the Czech Republic. In these examples we find that the skills necessary to lead a revolution aren't necessarily the same as those needed to lead a country.

How does this apply to health care? Seventy physician and nonphysician leaders attending a recent Medical Leadership Forum Conference were asked to prioritize major obstacles to the effectiveness of physicians in new leadership roles. "Lack of training or education on key knowledge, skills and attitudes needed for successful leadership" was near the top of the list. Not far from it was the observation: "Physicians feel under siege from all the changes . . . who to trust, who to partner with." And no wonder. Not only are we asking doctors to assume new roles for which they likely have received little training, we are asking them to assume roles diametrically opposite to those for which they have been trained.

Figure 12-1 lists some of the new leadership roles physicians are being asked to assume. Many of these require the types of orientation and skills listed in column 2 of figure 12-2, yet most M.D.'s have been trained or have learned to act in ways more characteristic of column 1, figure 12-2. A brief comparison of both columns reveals just how different they are.

Questions for Discussion

Review the material in figures 12-1 and 12-2 and answer the following questions:

1. What leadership roles do physicians hold in your health care organization?

FIGURE 12-1. Leadership Roles for Physicians

- CEO/COO
- Chief medical officer
- Vice president of medical affairs
- Clinical department chair
- President of medical staff
  —Committee chair
  —Clinical improvement team leader
  —Leader of a medical group practice

FIGURE 12-2. Differences between Physicians as Clinicians and Managers

Clinician	Manager
■ Autonomous	■ Collaborative
■ Patient oriented	■ Organization oriented
■ Empathic	■ Objective
■ Crisis oriented	■ Long-range planner
■ Quality focused	■ Cost focused
■ Doer	■ Delegator
■ Results oriented	■ Process oriented
■ Specialist	■ Generalist
■ Loyal to profession, peers	■ Loyal to organization
■ Linear thinker: left-brained	■ Creative, intuitive, right brained

Source: "The Unique Contribution of the Physician Executive to Health Care Management," New Leadership in Health Care Management: *The Physician Executive*, 1988.

2. What skills, experience, or attitudes do you feel are important to success in the leadership positions that you have identified?
3. What skills, experience, or other characteristics does your organization look for in filling its physician leadership positions?
4. Are doctors within the organization who are selected for leadership positions prepared in advance to assume their new role? If so, how?

Overcoming the Obstacles

In their new organizational leadership roles, physicians need a broad range of knowledge and skills. Many such skills are summarized in figure 12-3.

Doctors who want to acquire these skills often need flexible opportunities to do so, particularly if they need to continue their clinical practice. For some time, physician executives have been heavily used in managed care and academic

FIGURE 12-3. Leadership Knowledge and Skills

Knowledge: Understanding . . .

1. the industry: evolution of health care and health care delivery
2. organizations versus organisms
3. the change from individual patient–based to population-based health care delivery
4. how to balance efficiency and quality of care and align the incentives of everyone in the organization
5. the role, evaluation, acquisition, and use of information systems
6. continuous improvement theory and application
7. the fundamentals of business and finance: planning, marketing, finance and accounting, and performance evaluation
8. managed care: contracts, payment methods, network formation, and so on

Skills:

1. understanding and facilitating systems thinking
2. working in and through teams
3. decision making and leadership approaches and styles
4. conflict management
5. negotiation
6. change management
7. fostering continuous learning
8. creating continuous improvement systems
9. communication techniques
10. motivating and developing people

---

medical settings. Now they are increasingly sought after in other hospital settings as well as in for-profit companies.

Leadership responsibilities are becoming more demanding as well, sometimes necessitating a complete career change. According to a survey of 375 doctors by the Physician Executive Management Center in 1995, 87 percent of the respondents who held senior management positions had no clinical responsibilities.

How do doctors acquire the knowledge and skills they need in their new roles? One avenue is the American College of Physician Executives (ACPE), which had less than 1,000 members in the eight years following its inception in 1975. Today, ACPE has nearly 12,000 members, with a growth rate of 150 to 200 new members per month.

While traditional approaches to leadership development have focused on conferences, courses, or degree programs, newer options are emerging that not only provide for more flexibility, but emphasize use of real-world examples for problem solving and access to peers for support and networking.

Leadership Development Case Examples

Read the following case examples and answer the questions that follow.

Case 1

Mountain View Hospital was experiencing increasing tension in its relationships with doctors, largely because the hospital had begun purchasing selected physician practices. Management recognized that it could not afford continuing ill will for two reasons:

1. Competitors were courting the same physician practices that Mountain View wanted to acquire.
2. The hospital's strategic plan called for development of a physician-hospital organization (PHO), management services organization (MSO), and other collaborative initiatives with doctors that depended on identification of mutual goals and a willingness to work together.

Because the hospital needed to repair and strengthen its relationships with physicians and because it was planning a variety of initiatives that would require increased staffing, management created the position of vice president of medical affairs. This position would be responsible for overall hospital-doctor relations, practice acquisitions, PHO and MSO development, medical staff liaison activities, creation of a primary care network, recruitment and retention of new physicians, and physician leadership development.

Because improving the existing relationships with doctors was a major goal, it was determined that the person who would fill the vice president position needed to be a doctor, have credibility with peers, have been a successful clinician in his or her own practice, and have some prior leadership training or experience. A respected specialist who had recently sold his practice and had served five years ago as chief of staff was selected for the position with the understanding that additional leadership training would be available to him on a "learn-as-you-go" basis.

The vice president was given the opportunity to attend business courses offered at the local college or to attend a three-week intensive institute covering the fundamentals of management. The hospital would reimburse tuition and expenses as incurred.

Case 2

As part of a corporation-wide effort aimed at reevaluating and improving all of its leadership processes and structures, General Health System determined that one of its most important goals was to increase physician involvement in all levels of management and leadership throughout the system. To that end, a work group of board members, doctors, and executives was formed to look at

- how physicians might want to or be able to assume greater leadership roles in the organization
- the types of knowledge and skills that leadership roles required
- what current or potential physician leadership talent existed within the organization
- what skills and talent might need to be acquired
- how best to gain needed skills and abilities to get the right doctors in the right leadership positions at the right time
- how to ensure that processes were in place to both develop new leaders and provide existing leaders with opportunities to grow and develop

One of the group's recommendations was to establish a physician leadership development program that would offer a variety of options for doctors who were interested in gaining leadership skills. The program would consist of

- on-site educational programs on health care issues and trends
- off-site conferences, workshops, and institutes on the health care field and skills needed to be effective leaders or executives
- access to degree programs in medical management or health administration
- access to ad hoc learning networks of doctors designed to share experiences, tools, and techniques to address specific management issues or challenges via conference call or video teleconference
- establishment of an on-site resource center containing written, audio, video, and interactive resources on leadership and management
- opportunities for site visits to organizations with successful management or leadership models to learn about best practices
- pairing of seasoned and new organizational leaders in mentoring relationships to exchange questions and answers and provide support for learning the organization's leadership styles and culture
- establishment of a leadership council for senior physician, governance, and executive leaders to meet together to evaluate emerging issues and trends, discuss their implications for General Health System, and recommend options for addressing them

The physician leadership program could be developed in a tracked fashion to allow doctors to move from one level to the next; selected doctors would be given the opportunity to participate at different levels. Key physician leaders would be targeted as part of this process and assisted to put together individual development plans that would

- identify key leadership responsibilities
- describe individual learning needs and styles
- refine learning needs and set objectives based on prior background and experience

- select the array of topics and learning approaches to best meet the individual's learning needs and style
- periodically reevaluate needs and set new goals

To support the program, the organization would annually set aside funds dedicated to physician leadership development.

Questions for Discussion

1. Which case example do you think offers the best approach to developing physician leaders? Why?
2. What opportunities for leadership development does your organization offer to physicians?
3. Which opportunities for physician leadership development outlined in the case examples might work well in your organization?
4. Who is responsible for physician leader identification and development in your organization?
5. What financial support does your organization provide to assist physician leaders in their development efforts?

Just as physician leaders are made, not born, effective leadership development doesn't happen in an ad hoc fashion; it takes planning, coordination, and ongoing support and evaluation. The following tips can help trustees and other leaders ensure a comprehensive, flexible, and meaningful approach to physician leadership development.

Tips for Building a Successful Physician Leadership Development Effort

- Ensure that physician leadership development is a key organizational priority.
- Assign responsibility for leadership development to a senior executive, such as the vice president for medical affairs or chief medical director.
- Develop a program that includes a variety of educational topics and learning approaches to offer maximum flexibility for doctors interested in gaining leadership

skills. This is especially important for younger doctors who may be balancing their interest in acquiring leadership skills with the demands of starting a practice or raising a family.

- Ensure that your organization offers opportunities for leadership development that are peer-based, focus on solutions to real problems, and include ideas and tools that can be easily applied in the daily leadership context.
- Establish a budget item or fund for leadership development that is renewed at least annually.
- Encourage and assist doctors to develop individualized learning plans that match needs with a variety of topics and educational formats.
- Involve doctors in planning and developing your education efforts to ensure they meet a broad scope of needs.
- Communicate early and often to doctors the range of opportunities available to them to gain leadership knowledge and skills. Remember to clarify the type of organizational support available to assist them.
- Encourage senior physician leaders to act as mentors or advisers to new leaders and actively involve them in identifying potential leaders and developing a succession plan to ensure an ongoing stream of effective physician leaders.
- Evaluate your leadership development efforts periodically to ensure they are relevant and take advantage of state-of-the-art opportunities.

A Self-Assessment Questionnaire

The following survey addresses the board's roles and responsibilities in ensuring their organization has a comprehensive physician leadership development effort. It can be used as a stand-alone survey, or as part of an overall board self-evaluation process.

Have each trustee independently and anonymously rate the board's performance on the issues covered by each of the following questions. Compile and analyze all responses and discuss them with the entire board. Pay particular attention to questions with significant variation in responses (where some trustees rate board performance high and some rate it low) and those with predominately negative responses.

Although self-assessment surveys such as this are typically used with the board alone, it may be beneficial to have other leaders complete it as well because of their important involvement in the physician leadership development effort.

1. Involving doctors in a variety of leadership positions throughout our organization is a priority.

   ❑ Strongly Agree   ❑ Agree
   ❑ Disagree   ❑ Strongly Disagree

2. Funds are dedicated annually to support leadership development.

   ❑ Strongly Agree   ❑ Agree
   ❑ Disagree   ❑ Strongly Disagree

3. We have a comprehensive leadership development program that offers flexible opportunities to gain knowledge and skills for both new and seasoned physician leaders.

   ❑ Strongly Agree   ❑ Agree
   ❑ Disagree   ❑ Strongly Disagree

4. The board is familiar with the variety of leadership positions that physicians hold throughout the organization and has the opportunity to interact with these doctors at meetings and educational and social events.

   ❑ Strongly Agree   ❑ Agree
   ❑ Disagree   ❑ Strongly Disagree

5. Trustees attend, as appropriate, medical staff executive committee meetings, PHO board meetings, or other activities to gain a better understanding of clinical leadership issues and the role of the physician leader.

   ❑ Strongly Agree   ❑ Agree
   ❑ Disagree   ❑ Strongly Disagree

6. There is a formal process for evaluating the performance of physician executives to ensure ongoing effectiveness and to identify new learning needs and skills.

   ❑ Strongly Agree   ❑ Agree
   ❑ Disagree   ❑ Strongly Disagree

7. The role of physician board members and other voluntary physician leaders is clearly specified and communicated to candidates prior to their accepting these positions.

❑ Strongly Agree   ❑ Agree
❑ Disagree   ❑ Strongly Disagree

8. We have a leader succession plan.

❑ Strongly Agree   ❑ Agree
❑ Disagree   ❑ Strongly Disagree

Conclusion

Effective physician leaders and leadership development programs are made, not born. Organizations that want to attract new leaders and create meaningful learning opportunities for them need to be sure they offer financial support; a menu of topics; and flexible options that combine traditional with peer-based, applications-oriented approaches. The use of individualized learning plans, mentoring relationships, and other techniques for both new and seasoned physician leaders can help the organization build a cadre of effective leaders for today and for the future. Trustees, by understanding physician leadership development needs and options, can play an important role in helping those doctors gain the skills and experience they need to be effective and in helping to integrate them as partners into the organization's leadership environment.

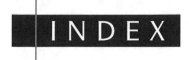

INDEX